DOCTOR SCHIFF'S ONE-DAY-AT-A-TIME WEIGHT-LOSS PLAN

"Dr. Martin Schiff's total mind-body plan has helped more than 75,000 patients lose weight *and keep it off*. His approach helps you recognize—and banish—the inner conflicts that cause overweight and learn to truly *enjoy* eating the delicious foods that slim you down but fill you with energy. No diets, no gimmicks... you savor one day at a time, as your spirits soar and your waistline shrinks."

—*The Literary Guild Magazine*

ALSO BY MARTIN M. SCHIFF, M.D.
Doctor Schiff's Miracle Weight-Loss Guide

DOCTOR SCHIFF'S ONE-DAY-AT-A-TIME WEIGHT-LOSS PLAN

Martin M. Schiff, M.D.

day books

A Division of STEIN AND DAY / *Publishers* / New York

FIRST DAY BOOKS EDITION 1982

First published in hardcover in 1980 by STEIN AND DAY/*Publishers*
Copyright © 1980 by Martin M. Schiff, M.D.
All rights reserved
Designed by David Miller
Printed in the United States of America
Stein and Day/*Publishers*
Scarborough House
Briarcliff Manor, N.Y. 10510

Library of Congress Cataloging in Publication Data

Schiff, Martin M. 1922–
  Doctor Schiff's One-day-at-a-time weight-loss plan.

  Includes index.
  1. Reducing—Psychological aspects. 2. Behavior modification. I. Title. II. Title: One-day-at-a-time weight-loss plan.
RM222.2.S269   613.2′5′01   79-5116
ISBN 0-8128-7048-4

To my loving wife Millie; our children Michael, David, Denise, and Howard; and our grandchildren Nicole and Robert

In loving memory of Celia and Irving Tepley

ACKNOWLEDGMENTS

To Bob Stone for his profound experience and superb craftsmanship. To Mort Dorchin for his timely, accurate guidance. To Patricia Day who applied the polish. To Bertha Camacho, my girl Friday. And to my patients who richly supply the ingredients that can benefit everyone.

PROLOGUE

Look to this day only—for yesterday is but a dream and tomorrow is merely a vision. But, this ONE DAY well-lived creates dreams of serenity, beauty, and happiness; also visions of love, success, and joy.

A picture is worth a thousand words.
A few well-chosen words and thoughts are worth a lifetime of understanding ... and happiness.

The inherent qualities of character and the fundamental human ingredients necessary to remain young in mind and in spirit are not diminished by the passage of time. They are regulated to a large degree by thoughts, emotions, feelings, and attitudes.

Thought is modified by the ability to utilize our basic intellect and senses, the capacity to "instruct" the mind to respond to our needs and wishes, the intensity of feeling, and the infinite power of stimulating the "inner being" to renew our enthusiasm for living day by day.

Old age is related to chronological age. It is also proportionate to the capacity and the desire to enjoy life to the fullest plus a willingness to develop and maintain cherished ideals and aspirations.

Physical changes are inevitable and occur spontaneously as we grow older. However, the spirit and the psyche are influenced by our "inner being" and consciousness.

Negative, unwanted and confused attitudes, emotions, and feelings increase the aging process—and not so incidentally our weight. Positive, happy, clear thoughts help perpetuate our youthful ways. . . . And these are slenderizing thoughts.

MARTIN SCHIFF, M.D., 1980

WHY YOU CAN LOSE WEIGHT PERMANENTLY ON THIS ONE-DAY-AT-A-TIME PLAN

When you go on this comprehensive, practical plan, the following discoveries and permanent changes eventually occur:

You lose weight and inches with ease day by day.

You feel better—both physically and mentally.

You function with more energy and enthusiasm, greater health and increased vitality.

You realize the plan is enlightening, effective, and gratifying.

You are attracted to nourishing, healthful foods.

You comprehend which emotions, feelings, thoughts, and attitudes you need to regulate and modify now and for the future.

You are highly motivated by good results to continue with the plan, repeating it one day at a time.

Each day on the plan reverses negative behavior patterns, and each repetition reinforces and enhances these behavioral changes.

You acquire insight and wisdom for living life without stress.

You eventually develop correct and improved eating and thinking habits, thus LOSING UNWANTED POUNDS PERMANENTLY.

CONTENTS

FOREWORD	13
I YOU EAT CORRECTLY ONE DAY AT A TIME	15
Why the One-Day-At-A-Time Plan Works	16
Mental Gymnastics or Physical Gymnastics—The Choice Is Yours	18
What You Can Eat on the One-Day-At-A-Time Plan	19
"I Feel So Good"	21
The Amazing Things You Find When You Take a Look Inside	22
The Secret of the One-Day-At-A-Time Plan	24
Live to Eat, or Eat to Live?	26
II YOU MAY NEVER HAVE TO REPEAT THE ONE-DAY-AT-A-TIME PLAN	28
The Many Faces of the Plan	30
Instead of Dieting, You Switch Foods on the Plan	32
The Two White Substances That Are Your Daily Poison	33
The Real Source of Eating Fun	35
Changes That Take Place	36
Getting to Know Yourself	38
What You Have Every Right to Expect from the Schiff Plan	40
Why You Don't Overeat and Regain in between Plan Days	41
III ALL THE DELICIOUS FOOD YOU CAN EAT ON THE ONE-DAY-AT-A-TIME PLAN	44
Here Is the Good News: This Is an Eating Program—Not a Non-Eating Program	46
Selections, One Day At A Time	50
Yesterday, Today, and Tomorrow	53
Say Goodbye to Your Old Self	56
Do Not Begin the One-Day-At-A-Time Plan Yet Because . . .	58

IV GROUND RULES FOR THE ONE DAY-AT-A-TIME PLAN — 61

Ground Rule Number One—No Willpower, No Trying	62
Don't Count Calories, Count "Kiks"	62
Substitute Quality for Quantity	64
Ground Rule Number Four—The Startling "Rule Of Two"	65
How to Act Like a Slender Person and Hasten That Day	68
An Unexpected Daily Source of Fat	69
The Unexpected Benefits That Come with Weight Loss, And Sooner Than You Think	70
How Writing Makes Things Right, Especially Weight	72

V ALTERNATIVE DAYS FOR EATING WELL ON THE PLAN — 76

Sugar Is Public Enemy No. 1	76
White Flour Is Public Enemy No. 2	78
Selecting Foods for Enjoyment, Nutrition, and Weight Loss	80
Ten Typical One-Day Menus	84
How and What to Switch to Increase the Fun	90
How to Derive More Satisfaction from Every Bite	91
How to Switch Mannerisms and Habits in Ways That Pay Off in Pounds Off	93

VI DOCTOR SCHIFF'S PRESCRIBED EATING DAY — 96

A Before-Breakfast Procedure That Helps Your Day Go Well	96
How to Start Diminishing Your Measurements	97
A Unique Way to Approach Your Meals This Day	98
How Recipes Add Joy and Subtract Pounds	100
Recipes That Add "Kiks" to Cooking and Dining As You Lose	101
Tips for Cooking to Lose Weight	118
Completing the One Day in a Special Way	120

VII THE AMAZING RULE OF TWO — 122

How to Extract Your Sweet Tooth	123
How the Two-Meal Person Can Easily Make It Four Meals	125
Changing Eating Times Gradually	128
The Three-Day Plan—One Day At A Time	130
Making a Meal out of Liquids	132

Contents

The Pure Protein Drink As an Extra Meal	133
A Word About Dietetic Foods	135
How to Experiment with Different Menu Plans Before Beginning the One-Day-At-A-Time Plan	136

VIII WHAT TO DO WHEN YOU ARE NOT ON THE PLAN TO KEEP THE POUNDS COMING OFF — 141

How to Identify Fattening Thoughts	142
Monitoring Fattening Thoughts One Day At A Time	147
Monitoring Techniques That Help Trap "Black Thoughts"	149
A Transformation Takes Place in Your Record of Thought Monitoring	150
You Begin to Lose Those Unwanted Pounds When You Pierce the Mental Armor	152
How the Power of Thought Shapes Our Ends	154

IX MENTAL INSTRUCTIONS THAT END FAULTY EATING AND THINKING HABITS PRACTICALLY OVERNIGHT — 158

Three Ways to Relax for Easy Learning Readiness	160
How to Give Mental "Instructions" That Change Eating Habits	162
Tips for Creating Eating Changes Mentally	165
Tips for Creating Higher Levels of Well-Being Mentally	167
Words and Pictures That Create a Slender Self-Image	169
Words and Pictures That Brighten Dismal Thoughts	170
Specific Instructions for Special Conditions	173

X ACCELERATING A NEW ATTRACTIVE LOOK — 175

Some Changes That Are About to Occur	176
How to Burn Off Pounds Without Exerting Yourself	178
How to Renew Weight Loss Once You Hit a Plateau	179
The Magic Formula for Continuing Weight Loss	181
How to Keep Problems from Triggering Appetite	184
How to Change the Subject and Change Yourself	186
Food as a Method of Self-Punishment	187
Emergency Measures That Deal Harshly with Fattening Foods and Fattening Thoughts	189
One Day At A Time Adds Up to Several Pounds Lost	191

XI SMALLER PORTIONS WITH A GREATER, ENJOYABLE TASTE	193
How to Make a Smaller Portion Just As Filling	194
Other Techniques for Losing Weight with Smaller Portions	196
Lose with Smaller Portions of This, Larger Portions of That	197
Sights and Sounds That Trigger False Hunger	199
Smaller Portions of Quality Protein Are Larger Portions of Nourishment	200
Instruct Your Mind to Make Smaller Portions Appear Larger	201
You Can Snack on the One-Day-At-A-Time Plan	203
Some Alternatives to the One-Day Plan	204
XII THE FIRST DAY OF THE REST OF YOUR FOREVER SLENDER LIFE	205
The Reward System for Changing Eating Habits	205
You Talk About Being Born Again	207
Fear of Failure Is Fattening	209
A Special "Accelerator" for Rapid Weight Loss	211
Protein Supplemental Plans	212
A Final Word About Weighty Problems	214
What to Do Before You Begin	216
The One-Day-At-A-Time Plan Begins—And Overweight Ends	217

Foreword

WHY THIS BOOK WILL WORK FOR YOU

I am a medical doctor. Eighteen of thirty years in my medical practice have been devoted to the specialty of bariatrics (weight control). I've helped thousands of patients lose weight and learn to lead a more enjoyable life on this One-Day-At-A-Time Plan.

It definitely *is not* a diet because eating correctly is only one of many factors required to achieve permanent and gratifying weight loss. However, "food for thought" plays a major role in this comprehensive and Holistic Weight-Loss Plan.

Dieting is a foolish game people play. It's like a grownup's "seesaw" or "yo-yo" game. You must recognize that this weight problem is multi-faceted; it is more than just food. See it as only a food problem and your weight may go down when on a diet, then rebound when you go off the diet.

With this Plan I help you to become aware of deeper thoughts, inner feelings, and subconscious programmings which are the actual underlying reasons for the overweight problem! You gain insight day-by-day. Gaining insight results in pounds lost—one day at a time, one ounce at a time.

Pounds drop away dramatically. It seems to be a miracle of the mind instead of the body. Actually it doesn't matter as you eventually become an attractive, contented, slender person.

Don't count calories. Don't buy special foods. Don't starve yourself time after time. Don't use gimmicks or fad diets—they don't work!

You don't have to play foolish games. But—you must learn to think, to understand, to enjoy, and to *do* for yourself.

Learning to change your mind and your life style day by day *is the key* to changing your eating habits and controlling your weight forever! Eventually, losing unwanted pounds permanently will become a joyous and miraculous breakthrough for YOU—out of the dreary dilemma of endless on again-off again dieting—into a bright, new, forever slender world.

DOCTOR SCHIFF'S
ONE-DAY-AT-A-TIME
WEIGHT-LOSS PLAN

YOU EAT CORRECTLY ONE DAY AT A TIME

"One day at a time, Doctor? How can anyone lose more than a pound or two? It seems impossible."

Yes, one day at a time.

Yes, a fraction of a pound up to one or two pounds is about all you are likely to lose during that one day. Perhaps three pounds at the most. It depends upon the amount of excess weight, food intake, exercise and physical activity, metabolism, body chemistry, constitutional differences, emotional and spiritual factors, life style, and so on.

No, it is not impossible to continue to lose weight. Remember the five minutes that you spent eating your first piece of layer cake and drinking your first soft drink? If I had told you then how many pounds those repeated five minutes or moments would eventually add to your body weight, you would have thought it impossible, too. This addition occurs day by day.

After reading this book, you will have a new eating plan for one day. It will be just as enjoyable as the cake and coke, but this time you will lose weight—and continue losing. Eventually, that one day can cause you to lose all the weight you need to shed for you to become more youthful, attractive, energetic. And it will all be as effortless as the cake and the coke.

Diets per se eventually fail because from a practical, emotional, and realistic viewpoint it is impossible to stay with a strict regime indefinitely. You are bound to yield to a tempting morsel "just this once." Those tempting morsels are ultimately self-defeating; thus the diet fails and you fail again. Continue to eat tempting morsels and eventually, one day at a time, you'll regain all the weight you had lost and maybe more.

You can have tempting morsels on this One-Day Plan, so you continue with it willingly and successfully. It takes willpower to go off this Plan, not to stay on it! It is effective and satisfying. *It definitely is not a diet.*

That's only part of the story. If I may get just a bit technical, let me explain the reason why my One-Day-At-A-Time Plan has slenderized thousands of women, men, teenagers, and children:

There are three basic approaches to weight loss—nutritional, behavioral, and analytical. The nutritionists honestly feel their method is the only one. The behaviorists are just as convinced their method is best. Of course, the therapists involved in the psychoanalytical method seldom talk to the other two.

The truth is, all three are correct when used together. Yet it is deplorable that all three go their own way with blinders on, not really caring about the other two methods.

Dr. Schiff's One-Day-At-A-Time Plan combines all three approaches. It is a comprehensive, permissive program based on correct food intake and nutrition, changed behavior, and a personal analysis of your own eating and thinking patterns. It is so effective and satisfying that *it is not really a diet.*

It is not my primary intention to describe the resulting permanent weight loss as a "miracle." I see it every day. Miracles are not supposed to be commonplace. But my slender patients who don't diet and still lose pound after pound insist, "It's a miracle!"

This "Miracle" is developed one day at a time. Some patients adopt the One-Day-at-a-Time Plan as a joyful way to eat day after day. Others repeat it occasionally, one day at a time.

Why the One-Day-at-a-Time Plan Works

New Yorker, Chicagoan, Angeleno, Walla Walla-an, anyone—you can enjoy and benefit from this book. After finishing it, you can then begin the One-Day Plan.

The "miracle" can then be yours: weight loss without tears, without unplanned, ineffective discipline, and without erroneous, illogical self-defeating willpower. Forever slender.

I am not talking only about the average overweight person. Yes, if you are 10, 20, 30, 40, or 50 pounds overweight, prepare for that one day which is going to change your life. But even if you are a superheavy weight, that one day will work for you—*if you* will work. In fact, it could be easier to lose 100 to 150 pounds than those pesky 10 pounds of unwanted padding.

You hear about people with some strange eating habits and experiences in this field. One woman on a supervised strict regimen volunteered to help some needy children. She convinced a local pastry shop to donate 12 dozen doughnuts to a party for the kids. She picked them up but the doughnuts never arrived at the party. She ate all 144.

This was an emotionally ill woman. Her illness was physical but it was caused by distorted, overwhelming mental factors (disturbed thoughts, distressed feelings).

You *cannot* divorce the mind from the body.

The mind can make you ill, and the mind can make you well. The mind can make you fat, and the mind can make you thin. *That is why, in order to be successful, a weight-control program needs to be mind-body oriented.* It needs to recognize both sides of the overweight problem—both the outside *and* the inside.

This weight-loss program does exactly that. That is why it works easily and fast, while others fail with much effort, time, and energy lost. Diet programs that do not recognize that you are a person, not just a body, are short-changing you. Don't sell yourself short.

There are two aspects to the weight problem:
1—Physical weight
2—Mental weight

You can cut out calories by sheer stubborn heroics for just so long. Then *you* cut out.

There is no starvation on my program. There is no deprivation either. If you feel anything less than full enjoyment with all your meals even for one day, then somewhere our communications have failed.

This One-Day-At-A-Time Plan works because it is you-oriented. Changes take place in *you* during that day. You enjoy those changes. You don't want them to stop happening. You also enjoy the food. So it is plain selfish pleasure either to stay on the plan or to repeat it again, soon.

Something else happens that is going to intrigue and help you.

Mental Gymnastics or Physical Gymnastics—
The Choice Is Yours

Let me open my records and tell you about the case of Lori H. (All names I use in this book are changed to hide the identity of the patient because it gets really personal—as personal as you can get.)

"High blood pressure is a second cousin to obesity." I looked knowingly into the blue eyes of Lori, one of a score of patients attending my five-hour orientation lecture. This book is basically that lecture.

I knew Mrs. H.'s blood pressure to be 182 over 104. Exactly 198½ pounds ballooned on her five foot six frame. She was in for some health problems—with an overworked heart the greatest risk.

After the lecture, she waited to talk to me. "It sounds so easy," she exclaimed, "I can't wait to begin."

"Then why wait. Begin now. It does not have to wait for a meal. Begin to think about your eating ways as you walk out the door—how, what, when, where, why."

She nodded enthusiastically and left.

I did not see her again until September, four months later. In those few months she lost 30 pounds. But even better news, her blood pressure dropped to 124 over 88, within normal brackets for her 35 years. I also noted that while her pulse had been recorded as 102 during the first visit, it too was a more normal 84.

"Remember, Doctor Schiff, you asked me to think about my eating habits when I left your office. Well, I haven't stopped. The next day, I went strictly by the book, eating only from the groups on your permitted food list. As I recall I made beef stew with onions, carrots, and lean beef. I don't remember what foods I ate, except there was an abundance and variety of delicious foods, mostly protein. I lost three pounds the first day."

Lori H. went on to explain how her "mental gymnastics" helped—how she kept looking for clues during the day that would ordinarily drive her to the refrigerator. "I love ice cream," popped into her mind. She popped it right out, substituting, "I think about, understand, and love myself."

"I became more interested in myself than in food. Then without thinking, I ate only permitted foods and followed the program."

I've lost count of how many Lori H.'s I know. Thousands of my patients have acquired the ability to "set their mind" for a diet, then, be on a conscious diet for one day; then not be on a diet consciously at all. Almost before realizing, they learn to eat correctly—one day at a time.

This particular Lori H. had returned in order to reinforce her new method of eating with self-awareness. We discussed her new insight into herself.

"Before, when I saw heavy people, I was disgusted. I realized I looked like them. I made a judgment about myself. Now they do not remind me of me. I am in control. This reduces my anxiety. I don't smother emotional upsets with food. I think about, understand, and do for myself—I love myself."

She described her success as if her life depended upon it. It did.

You could say that Lori H. did some mental gymnastics. They are easy and fun. More fun than physical gymnastics. Do you know how much physical exercise it takes to lose a pound? Well, if you weighed 200 pounds, to lose just one pound, you would have to:

Run very fast for 3½ hours, or
Run moderately fast for 4½ hours, or
Exercise strenuously for 4 hours, or
Walk moderately fast for 8½ hours.

Which would you prefer to do?:
  (a) Strenuous physical exercise for four hours to lose one pound, or
  (b) Daydream-type mental gymnastics for a few minutes to lose pound after pound.

Mental gymnastics pay off in easy weight loss. Take my advice: choose (b).

What You Can Eat on the One-Day-At-A-Time Plan

Let's get down to the "meat" of the One-Day-At-A-Time program—and there's plenty of that. Included also are many delicious foods that you are enjoying now.

The key to this very important one day is not primarily the foods you eat; it's what you do not eat. On the pages ahead I will give you a list of allowed foods. You will select those you enjoy the most and create your own menus.

Natalie F. is eating breakfast on the One-Day-At-A-Time Plan. Yesterday, before the plan, she had a ham omelet, hash brown potatoes, toast, coffee. Today, she is having an omelet again. This time a spinach omelet. No toast and potatoes. She has switched to low-fat cottage cheese, and treated herself to a second cup of coffee, without cream and sugar.

Yesterday, she was not on the One-Day-At-A-Time Plan. For lunch she had broiled halibut, potatoes, and string beans. Today, she is on the program. She finished the leftover halibut and string beans but skipped the potatoes. Instead, she has a portion of spinach left over from this morning's omelet. Yesterday's dinner: Mexican chile and tortillas. Today's One-Day-At-A-Time Plan dinner: old-fashioned boiled beef and fresh vegetables. As a late snack she has a piece of cheese and a cup of tea with lemon only.

Natalie F. felt so good after this one day that she decided to eliminate potatoes and Mexican beans and corn from her meals. She decided also to omit toast in the morning. "If that's all it takes to feel so good, goodbye bread and potatoes. They give me less pleasure than I get from doing without them." She went from 156 pounds to 132 pounds between March 15 and June 7.

"Natalie, how many times did you repeat the one day of diet during this period?" I asked.

"Never, really, doctor," she replied. "I just naturally know what I need to eat to feel as though I'm standing on top of the world—it's as though I'm not on a diet!"

The foods you eat on the One-Day-At-A-Time Plan are the food you eat now, with few exceptions. But each of these exceptions is a key pound-maker. And there is always another good food to substitute in its place. So it is *not* a diet. It is a planned substitution.

The more imaginative you are with the foods you switch, the more you will enjoy the one day of planned, correct, and improved eating. By that I mean: like something and you repeat it. *Repeat it, and it soon becomes a habit. We make ourselves "creatures of habit."*

Bread and potatoes may be a habit with you right now. Soon, after you finish reading this book and begin the One-Day-At-A-Time approach, fish may become a habit with you. You may want sardines for breakfast, tuna salad for lunch, and broiled salmon almondine for dinner. Or you may get hooked on low-fat cottage cheese or low-fat yogurt, or become a devotee of omelets in their infinite variety or of chopped steak with onions or with peppers or with mushrooms or with . . .

You are substituting one habit for another—a slenderizing, joyful habit for a fattening, joyless habit.

The fattening habit started in the past. The slenderizing habit is about to start.

"I Feel So Good!"

If you have been on a typical calorie-counting diet, you know what it is like. You are depleted, discontented, and eventually disillusioned. All the great expectations go down as you experience the negative, joyless feelings—for as long as you can take them.

Then your weight goes back up.

Those who have been on the One-Day-At-A-Time Plan don't experience these negative feelings. Instead, they feel rejuvenated, satisfied, joyful. It's almost like being on a "high."

Such feelings *demand* repeating. And that is exactly what happens. Some repeat the one day once a week. They pick a day such as Monday, and every Monday they repeat the One-Day-At-A-Time Plan. That seems to be a favorite day—after weekend gustatorial festivities.

Others repeat the One Day whenever the spirit, or scale, moves them. Still others make it their "habitual" way of improved eating.

My words don't count as much as my patients' words.

Kathleen H. writes, "I feel *stronger* than ever. What is giving me the strength . . . is the image of the new me."

"I like myself more," writes June V., "I look better and have more of an outgoing, bubbly personality. I have increased self-confidence and am able to express my inner feelings outwardly."

A month earlier, soon after starting on the program, June noted the following eight benefits: "1. Look better; 2. Feel better; 3. Weigh less; 4. No more sleepless nights (a miracle); 5. No pain from an old operation incision; 6. Overweight neighbors are jealous; 7. Pain in the knees is gone; 8. Even my husband looks and feels better."

Writes Mary P., "I weighed only 147 when I had my second baby; thanks to you, I did not stuff myself. I really felt great. People told me how good I looked. I was back on my feet soon after the baby was born; even surprised my doctor."

Susann L., 50, has a different life style, different benefits. "What has happened to me on this program has been amazing. I have been on and off diets for 25 years. I was very unhappy. I saw myself old, sick, and ugly. Now my outlook on life is so beautiful. I experience love and emotions I never knew before. I have been born again. I work eight hours a day and am less tired than younger people who work with me and eat junk food."

Anita C., 24, tells me, "You've made me feel important within myself. . . . I'm giving more of myself on the job . . . I have much more energy. Diets leave me depressed, frustrated, disgusted, and always down in the dumps. . . . My husband is so thrilled with the new me . . . I know I'll never be fat again."

The Amazing Things You Find When You Take a Look Inside

Our brain is like a computer. It runs our body automatically without our having to give a single conscious thought to moving our lungs, beating our heart, squeezing our glands, or filtering chemicals with our kidneys.

It is all automatic. They say we are born with some two thousand "instructions" that enable these automatic processes to function as nature intended. Two of these are hunger when we need food and thirst when we need water.

However, when mother rewards a child for good behavior with ice cream or candy, a new "instruction" is added: ice cream equals mother love. We all need mother's love a lot more than we need ice cream, but because the two have become equated—much the way Pavlov's dogs "learned" to make their saliva flow at the sound of a bell when bells rang as food was given to them—"ice cream bells" ring for us constantly.

Take Marsha W., 39, divorced, an office worker with three children. During her three years of marital problems, she drank wine

You Eat Correctly One Day At A Time

at home "until I was numb." This numbness was like a sedative to insulate her from her husband's irritating behavior.

After her divorce, the children fought constantly, causing more irritation, more thirst for wine. The first thing she did when she went home was to pour herself a tall glass of wine so she would be "ready."

The more wine she drank, the more she thought she was able to cope with her problems and her children. And the closer she came to being an alcoholic and a weight-aholic.

When she visited my office she weighed 132, which was too much for her five foot one frame. Within six weeks she was down to 120 with hardly any changes in her eating habits and only one change in her drinking habit. I taught her how to reprogram ("instruct") the mind back to its natural state: water satisfies thirst.

She did this well. She fixed herself a tall glass of ice water whenever she felt the desire for wine. She sometimes had three or four of these during an evening. She felt better, looked better, and for some strange reason, the children began to behave better.

There are many serious problems, confused thoughts, and disturbed or negative emotions in our lives that create false hunger (appetite) and false thirst. Loneliness, feelings of inadequacy, depression, boredom, frustrations, disgust, and the like—all do it, *only* if we allow it.

Many a woman has an unreal "love affair" going with her refrigerator. Many a man is giving himself an unreal "promotion" with two martinis—or more. Many a teenager is finding unreal "scholastic acceptance" in a bottle of coke or some other junk food.

Added to these inner "instructions" are the outer pressures:

"You are too thin. You should eat more."

"Have you tried the new pizza place yet?"

"Wanna drink?—Don't be a party pooper."

"They have a new flavor at Don's Ice Cream Parlor."

"Don't leave food on your plate. Think of all the starving people in the world."

"Have a bite, it won't hurt."

"Have another portion—I made it myself."

Could you add to this list?

When we take a look inside, we usually discover some amazing things about ourselves. We find that we are "conditioned" or "programmed." We find that it is not our physical glands that are making us overeat, but our mental gleanings—input we have accepted as "instructions." We eat and drink when we are not actually hungry or thirsty.

When we look inside we learn how the fat between our ears deposits fat between our ribs—and thighs and hips and arms. Get the picture?

The Secret of the One-Day-At-A-Time Plan

A six footer came into my office. He was immense. Leonard J., 37, weighed 317 pounds and was unemployed. He had been to several doctors who had tried various medications and diets, but Lenny continued to gain weight.

I saw Lenny once a month for two months, then I did not see him until nearly a year later. In eleven months he had lost 76 pounds. Also his blood pressure dropped 30 points.

He told me how he had been changed by the program. "It helped me to unscrew my head. Now I live one day at a time. I am in control of my food intake. It has been a gradual process, but it never seemed to me that I was on a diet at any time. I simply follow the food guide. This is so easy compared to other diets I have been on, I don't consider it a diet.

"Actually I follow the Plan's food guide only one day a month. But I have also cut down drastically on quantity and don't eat junk food. I 'prove' I can do it."

He explained how he had found a job, due largely to his weight loss, and was deriving a lot more "fun out of life." He said his goal was to go below 200 pounds. He's probably there by now—eating correctly only one day a month.

The key lies in what Leonard J. said: "I'm getting a lot more fun out of life."

The secret underlying the success of the program is extracting more fun out of life.

"The old clothes form is an unsightly thing in the closet . . . from a size twenty to a fourteen . . . hiking and swimming again." Certainly this 65-year-old woman, Mrs. Elizabeth G., who went from 200 pounds to 162 in nine months, is now having more fun.

You Eat Correctly One Day At A Time

"In my vocation as an actress, I have found new freedom, poise, and power previously stifled by the physical weight and the emotional weight."

Nancy H., 32, is having more fun at 139 pounds in October than at 203 pounds the previous March. "I like myself," she says, "and for the first time in my life, I have a sense of my own worth."

When Doris F., 24, came to my office for the first time she weighed 158. Picture a beautiful face and a radiant complexion on a buxom body. It was like the moon coming over the mountain.

Doris had problems. But they were very personal to her and she did not want to admit to herself that she had any. She went on the physical and eating aspects of the program. Within eight months, no more mountain. She had glided down to 130. When she stepped off the scale, she looked glum.

"I'm faking it, Dr. Schiff."

"You can't fool the scale," I replied.

I did not know exactly what she meant until the next visit. She was up to 154 again. The moon was full.

"See what I mean?"

"I see what I see. Suppose you tell me what it means."

Thereupon followed a confession. She said she had a "trouble zone." She could not even name it for herself, much less for me. Whenever the "trouble zone" surfaced, she would eat. "As I eat I go into a sort of trance. I don't even think about the 'trouble zone.' What a perfect escape!"

I did not want to push her into baring her troubles to me, but I encouraged her to think more about them herself. "Writing helps thinking," I explained, "Write to yourself—write about your troubles and yourself."

She did. She analyzed her problem. She thought about herself. Instead of turning her back on her problem and opening her mouth to food, she jumped right into the problem situation. "I found a way out—fat was my loophole. Now I'm learning not to feel sorry for myself. I'm learning a happier, brighter approach to *me*. . . . It is a one-day-at-a-time process. I concern myself with doing the best I can today, at this moment. . . . It makes the program exciting for me. Day by day, pound by pound, thought by thought, action by action."

Doris emerged as a slender, beautiful, happy person. No moon, and plenty of sunlight.

In this weight program, you learn to know yourself better. You begin to live your life more fully. You lose weight. You enjoy. And that spells fun.

Live to Eat, or Eat to Live?

When you let life's problems "bug" you, you are not extracting the fun you deserve out of life. So you seek to derive that fun from food. Living to have fun becomes living to eat. However, living to eat is an error.

What you are actually doing is teaching yourself to eat, eat, eat. Other original, natural programmings "move over" to accommodate this new learning process (this new game). Your lungs continue to breathe although each breath does less and less for each cell as the fat cells multiply. As your body builds more blood capillaries to reach the new fat, the heart pumps harder to reach these new areas, and the blood pressure builds up.

As your fun continues to be food, your body continues to adjust to this foolish game. It's rough on your heart and other vital organs. They were designed to function under different conditions. Then one day, an organ stops functioning. It's the end of the game, the end of the fun.

You can reverse this process so easily. It started imperceptibly. It can end imperceptibly. It can end, and a new slender life can begin— all in one day.

A person is both mind and body. It's a *good* bet that an overweight person has as much fat between the ears as over the rest of his or her body. You cannot successfully help an overweight person via the body alone any more than you can make the left side thin while the right side stays padded.

To change from a "live to eat" to an "eat to live" person once again takes mind-body teamwork. That teamwork changes the whole diet concept. It no longer requires endless weeks or months of strenuous dieting. One day can cause the "eat to live" approach to begin working immediately.

I have seen marriages on the rocks become marriages on feather beds. I have seen businesses on the rocks begin to flow with profit. I have seen men and women in the depths of despair begin to flower with the joy of life. I have seen hopeless, frustrated, obese patients shed the mantle of their fatty armor and become their slender, youthful selves again.

I offer this to you.

11

YOU MAY NEVER HAVE TO REPEAT THE ONE-DAY-AT-A-TIME PLAN

"My husband left me alone sexually. He said I did not appeal to him. 'Look in the mirror,' he said, 'see how fat you've become and you'll see why I don't want to touch you.' This depressed me, so I stuffed myself with food."

The lack of sexual fulfillment is often in the forefront as a manipulator of taste buds.

This happens to be Susan K., 42, talking. She is five three, weighs 150. She ate the following the day before yesterday:

Breakfast:	Orange juice Pancakes with syrup Coffee with sugar and cream
Mid-morning:	Doughnut Coffee with sugar and cream
Lunch:	Club sandwich Potato salad
Mid-afternoon:	Slices of meat Bread
Dinner:	Roast beef Roast potatoes Vegetable Wine Fruit Coffee with sugar and cream
Late evening:	Cornflakes with milk, sugar

You May Never Have to Repeat the One-Day-At-A-Time Plan

Susan then began my weight-control plan. She attended the initial orientation meeting.

This is what Susan ate today:

Breakfast:	Seafood omelet Coffee without cream or sugar
Mid-morning:	V-8 juice
Lunch:	Liver and onions String beans Iced tea with lemon only
Mid-afternoon:	Slices of bell peppers filled with cottage cheese
Dinner:	T-bone steak Carrots Cole slaw Gelatin dessert Coffee—black, no sugar
Late evening:	Sliced cheese Herb tea

Susan had never combined seafood and eggs in an omelet. She loved it. Lunch was a treat, liver and onions being a favorite of hers. What more could she ask for dinner than a steak with all the trimmings plus dessert. And in between these three square meals, she had three mini-meals—a morning, afternoon, and evening snack.

What has all this food to do with Susan's problem with her husband?

Well, Susan's problem with her husband was not new. He had been nastily criticizing her excessive weight for years. She had tried every diet under the sun—and failed. Even the Weight Watchers could not bear watching her weight anymore.

The Schiff Plan could have been the whole trip all over again. But it wasn't. A new dimension had been added—awareness of the connection between food and sex. It developed from the self-awareness encouraged on the plan. And her statements stem from this self-awareness.

She had fun on her "one day." Later she found herself making her week's shopping list from the allowed foods of the One-Day-At-A-Time program. Soon she automatically favored those foods when dining out. She became more a gourmet than a gourmand, and her dining experiences became more enjoyable and slenderizing.

"I can see a new confidence building in me daily as I learn to think about, understand, and love myself," she told me. "I find myself asserting my opinions more at home. I have developed more self-confidence. Also, I am more demanding. If I feel I need something, I get it."

Susan became a youthful, attractive 114-pound brunette. But her sexual relations problem with her husband was not solved. Her husband did not change in the new situation. "I discovered it was my husband who had the problem all along. He claims he tries, but now he is too tired."

A short time later, they were divorced, and Susan started a new life in another state. It really was a new life—because it was a new Susan.

The Many Faces of the Plan

Margaret C., 49, five foot four and a roly poly 203 pounds, started the program.

A few weeks later she related what happened after only a few days. "I was feeling hungry when I remembered something you said: hunger is frequently thirst. So I opened the refrigerator and had a large glass of cold water instead. To my surprise, this is what I really wanted."

For years diets have come and gone. Usually they have been described by their predominant characteristic: the grapefruit diet, the rice diet, the low-carbohydrate diet, the drinking man's diet, the egg diet, and so on.

The One-Day-At-A-Time method has so many good points going for it that there is no one peg upon which to hang it.

1. The allowed foods are low-carbohydrate, low-fat foods. But it

You May Never Have to Repeat the One-Day-At-A-Time Plan 31

would be wrong to tell anyone that the One-Day-At-A-Time method is "a low-carbohydrate, low-fat program." It is not. First, it is too permissive to rate as a stringent program, such as the name indicates. Second, there is so much more than food involved in the Plan or Program.

2. Through this book, I am better able to communicate with your mind and start you on a comprehensive, total, and effective program. This is so important that I give you no rigid menus such as others do—first day, second day, third day, etc. There is only One Day, thanks to the mind-body partnership.

3. Good nutrition is part of the plan. You need to feed every cell in your body, plan or no plan. Many overweight people are actually undernourished. You cannot have balanced nutrition on a starvation or carrot stick diet. As a doctor, your health is my primary concern. Still, as balanced as the One-Day-At-A-Time concept is, I recommend that you keep your family physician informed of your altered food intake.

4. You switch foods. You do not cut out or cut down drastically. If you decide to repeat the One-Day-At-A-Time procedure, it can be completely different and enjoyable every One Day.

5. You add meals. I heartily recommend meals in between meals. See my "Rule of Two" in Chapter VII.

6. Versatility. There is so much freedom (permissiveness) that even with thousands of people on this plan, I doubt if any two will ever choose the exact same menu for that One Day. In fact, the One-Day-At-A-Time Plan permits you to eat many things you now enjoy while eliminating many fattening foods. Now that's versatility. See Chapter X. You can even decide to go on the One-Day-At-A-Time Plan for two days, three days, or more. Many people repeat it or stay on it because they want to, not because they have to.

7. New mental "instructions" are another important factor that the One-Day-At-A-Time method has going for it. You have conditioned your mind and body to a certain way of thinking—a fattening way. It required no effort. You are overweight. You can now reverse the process. You can "instruct" your mind and body toward a different way of thinking—a slenderizing way. You lose weight. It takes no effort. Once you know the "trick" (it's in Chapter VIII), you'll be amazed how easy it is to teach your appetite to behave and to control your hunger.

8. Behavior modification, or forming new eating habits, is another important attribute. There are simple ways to serve your meals and operate your knife and fork to accelerate your transformation from a silhouette like this: "O", to a silhouette more like this: "I."

Instead of Dieting, You Switch Foods on the Plan

Mrs. Norah C., age 49, height five feet four inches, weight a chubby 178 pounds, came to the office for her initial visit in February, 1976.

An initial visit to my office is not a matter of 15 or 20 minutes. It requires five hours. Besides a brief interview and physical, people wanting to lose weight attend a five-hour orientation lecture in which I discuss roughly the same ground I cover in this book. So, in effect, Mrs. C. read this book before returning home to go on her One-Day-At-A-Time program.

I did not see her again until three months later. What a difference! Her weight was normal. She was a slim 129 pounds. She returned, she said, because she wanted to lose another 15 pounds and needed additional help.

"How come?" I asked. "You've done all right on your own so far."

"I guess just talking with you will help," she replied.

She went on to tell me how she eliminated all products with sugar or flour the day after her initial visit. "After hearing your talk, I realized those two ingredients had made me fat all my life."

It was a problem that very first day, she admitted. She especially missed her bread. However, she changed her thinking. Although she lost no weight that first day, she lost something more important—a daily penchant for bread and cookies. At the end of one week she had lost more than three pounds.

"By then I had reorganized my eating habits," she explained. "I was feeling good merely switching from high-fat, high-carbohydrate foods to high-protein foods. Thus, the new way of eating soon became natural for me. I discovered the right way of eating can become a habit, too, just as the wrong way had."

I assured her it could indeed.

Mrs. C. is continuing her new eating habits. All I did at the second visit was to suggest additional ways to become aware of her attitudes and reactions in her everyday activities. Also, she was weighing herself almost everyday. "Forget it," I told her. "Once a week is often enough. Tension about your progress can cause you to backslide." When she left she was all smiles. I have not seen her since. In fact, I think her second visit wasn't necessary. She had found the solution to her lifelong overweight problem that very first day.

I am now going to tell you about those two white substances—white flour and white sugar. If everyone switched these empty caloric ingredients out and protein foods in, bariatric (weight control) physicians would have to switch their specialty.

The Two White Substances That Are Your Daily Poison

There are no permitted foods on that One Day that contain white sugar or white flour. The very thought of white sugar repulses me. If someone forced you to eat a pound of white sugar, spoon after disgusting spoon, you would never want to face that white stuff again in your life.

White sugar is a killer. It is killing hundreds of thousands yearly! The medical records don't read "death due to sugar poisoning," but they really should. Instead, they read "heart failure," "cerebral-vascular failure," "kidney failure," "circulatory failure," "pulmonary failure," or many other failures—all induced by the side effects of sugar, the chief of which is *fat*.

Sugar is a carbohydrate. Carbohydrate is energy. We need energy. But, do we not need sugar?

There are carbohydrates in grains, dairy products, fruits, and vegetables. These are more desirable carbohydrates than white sugar because they contain other forms of nourishment: minerals and vitamins and proteins.

Sugar—white especially—contains empty carbohydrates. No nourishment. In fact, studies show sugar leaches important minerals from our body. It also stimulates the pancreas excessively to produce too much insulin. This can cause fatigue or blackouts. Sugar can lead to tooth decay. Its high calorie count provides more energy than we can burn. Results: it burdens our vital organs with a fat load.

White flour is carbohydrate. We need it like we need white sugar. Grain is excellent food. But man takes the grain and hulls it, denudes it, pounds it, and extracts all the good from it so it won't spoil. Even worms know there's no real food in white flour.

White sugar and white flour find their way into every nook, shelf, case, and cranny of the food store. Sugar is in canned vegetables and canned fruits, dry cereal, and most prepared foods. Read the fine print. You'll see. Sugar added. It is in candy, ice cream, and soft drinks where all can see, but it hides in many other foods where you'd least expect it.

White flour is king of the fast foods. Take a look at all of these baked goods—bread, rolls, doughs, pastry, cookies, cakes, pies. Here king white flour teams up with queen sugar to proliferate pounds on you. Then there are the pancake mixes, the waffles, the spaghetti, macaroni, and other pastas. Not an ounce of real food in a carload. There exists a whole world of delicious foods without these two fatteners.

Look at the two right now: white sugar, white flour. See them as your private enemies number 1 and 2. They also happen to be public enemies, but we are interested in you. See them as personal enemies to you. Dangerous enemies. Hit men with a contract out for you.

Let there be no mistake about it. *Sugar and flour are the chief contributors to obesity, and obesity is a health menace of major proportions.* It increases your chances of becoming ill and then developing complications. It diminishes your ability to respond to treatment. If it does not "get you" today, it "gets you" tomorrow.

You can escape these enemies—white sugar and white flour. Just substitute other more nourishing sweeteners, other more nourishing grains in their place. And I might add, less fattening too.

I am going to help you to do this in the pages ahead. I'll help you to eat lustier meals than ever before, without white poison in it. And thirst-quenching drinks, such as Dr. Schiff's Protein Punch, Dr. Schiff's Energy Sling, and Dr. Schiff's Screwdriver, Thin Fizz, and Highball. I want you to have fun on Day One. And there is a lot more low-calorie eating fun than is to be found in white sugar and white flour.

The Real Source of Eating Fun

Protein foods are the mainstay of most successful weight-loss methods. If you were to take the water out of a human body, then slice away the stored-up unneeded fat, the rest would be more than 90 percent protein.

Since we are mostly protein, we need to eat protein. Adding to this important fact is the point that although our body can convert fats, carbohydrates, and protein into energy, it cannot convert anything into protein. Fats and carbohydrates cannot be converted into protein. Little wonder that extremely low-calorie diets which are also low in protein hurt. Besides starving us, they deprive every cell in our body of needed nourishment.

The Plan's food components emphasize proteins and de-emphasize fats and carbohydrates. The way I help you know the difference is to give you a list of preferred foods and a list of banned foods. On the preferred foods is a parade of proteins. Just reading the list (in the next chapter) will make your mouth water.

Are proteins more expensive than other foods? Here's what Bill H., 32, says: "We cut our grocery bill by 50 to 75 dollars a month buying the right food instead of junk. And it is better quality food."

Protein food helped bring Bill's weight down from 245 pounds on June 3rd to 185 pounds two months later on August 5th—a proper weight for his six foot two height.

Add to the figure on the check-out counter cash register the doctor's bills that are caused from buying "convenience" foods. Precooked carrots with sugar. Prebaked apple pie with sugar and white flour. Quick and easy. A quick way to fatten and an easy way to shorten your life.

Protein is another story. It slenderizes. It energizes. It heals. It builds body tissue. It adds life.

Violet F. likes cheese. It is high in protein. It likes her. She chose a Sunday for her first day on the One-Day-At-A-Time method. This is what she ate:

8:30 a.m.:   1 Hard-boiled egg
              ½ Cup Cottage cheese
              ½ Cup Homemade fruit sauce

10:00 a.m.:	2 Slices of Gouda cheese Coffee, black
2:30 p.m.:	2 oz. Chopped sirloin of beef patty with chopped onions 2 Scrambled eggs Fresh vegetable salad Coffee, black
4:00 p.m.	Diet soda
6:30 p.m.:	Celery and carrot sticks 2 oz. Mozzarella cheese ½ Cup Cottage cheese mixed with freshly sauteed mushrooms 1 Fruit Coffee, black

The point: protein, fruit, vegetables equal good nutrition—both a balanced, healthy intake and permissive.

Violet did not have a single guilty moment on that One-Day method by eating cheese three or four times a day. It is mostly protein, especially the cheeses she chose. In fact, Violet's menu was predominantly protein. She ate well. Yet she lost a pound.

Violet did more than eat well. She drank six glasses of water. She kept a record of her food and beverage intake. She noted when she was hungry and her feelings at those times. She thought about herself. She pondered. She relaxed. That one-day event made more than a one-pound difference in Violet's life.

Protein is an important ingredient in the Plan, but all the other aspects of the weight-loss program are extremely important, too.

Changes That Take Place

The beginning of weight loss.
The beginning of self-awareness.
The beginning of confidence.
The beginning of self-understanding.

These are the outward accomplishments on the One-Day-At-A-Time Plan.

But there are also inner changes that take place. These inner changes promote continued weight loss, continued self-awareness, continued confidence, and continued self-understanding.

It is as though a change of polarity has occurred on that one day—from negative to positive. On the negative side: weight gain, thoughtless eating, feelings of failure. On the positive side: weight loss, a new interest in self, visions of success.

All in one day, you ask?

All in one minute, I reply.

It takes longer than a minute to read this book. It takes longer than a minute to prepare for the One-Day-At-A-Time Plan. It takes longer than a minute to eat your way through that One Day.

But all it requires is one minute, maybe less, for the change of polarity to take place mentally that produces a change of polarity physically.

The mental change begins with a decision. The decision triggers a physical change. Your body actually begins to function differently hours before you eat your first meal on the One-Day-At-A-Time Plan. It is a very real, metabolic change. It is as if the army has received new orders. "Weight loss alert! Prepare to reverse storage process!"

The body is shaped by the mind. You can sense what a person is like, when you first meet, by the person's appearance. The consciousness (mind) we have is related closely to the body we have. Change one, you change the other.

You are about to change your mind. You are going to decide that you will be more self-conscious, and by so being, you can become slender and attractive at any age without the yo-yo ups and downs of heartbreaking diets. That change of mind is going to cause a change of body. That change occurs day by day, one moment at a time.

It may be subtle at first—subtle changes in psychological functioning which in turn affect feelings and appetites, subtle changes in metabolism, subtle changes in body chemistry, subtle changes in weight and body contour.

All this will take place before you are through reading this book. A subtle change in you.

Getting to Know Yourself

There are clinics in large cities devoted to self-help and self-understanding. They often utilize hypnotism and self-hypnotism, but these terms are beginning to be recognized as special techniques of the larger process for reconditioning or reprogramming, that is "instructing" the mind. Old cause-effect relationships are disconnected, and new cause-effect relationships are then established in their place.

If you were to observe the activities at such a clinic, you would see the patient relaxing in a comfortable living-room-like office. The therapist might be helping with monotonous sounds or changing lights, or demonstrating muscle relaxing techniques.

Then the therapist would give the patient "instructions." These instructions would be strange because the therapist would sound as if the patient had control over uncontrollable mind and body functions. He might be saying such things as:

"You are satisfied with smaller portions."

"You find that ice cream tastes like castor oil."

"By taking a deep breath, in between meals, hunger disappears."

"By learning to relax, you will help yourself to shed some pounds."

He is not talking to the person's conscious mind. He is actually "instructing" the person's subconscious mind—the part of the mind that runs the body.

When the patient leaves, he does not have to diet. He automatically eats the nonfattening foods. You could call this the "No Day Plan."

We do not use hypnotism or self-hypnotism in this One-Day-At-A-Time approach. But we do reach the subconscious mind. We "instruct" it. We teach it new reactions, new cause-effect relationships.

Lonely equals chocolate bar. Depressed equals layer cake. Frustrated equals ice cream. Nervousness equals snacks. And so on, and so on. These are the typical old "instructions" in the subconscious mind that we cancel and eliminate.

We then connect loneliness, depression, frustration, nervousness, and other false, fattening appetite causes to new, slenderizing and different nonfood or allowable food effects. It is better to eat a few slices of cheese, a chicken leg, an allowable dessert, or the like, than to eat a piece of pie with ice cream. It's that simple.

We must use relaxation. *Relaxation is the "doorway" to the subconscious mind.* The doorway may be labeled self-hypnotism but it still requires relaxation. It may be labeled meditation but it still requires relaxation. It may be labeled psycho-synthesis, Mind Control, yoga, or any number of disciplines, but they all require relaxation. When we relax and give ourselves "mental instructions," those instructions are accepted by the subconscious mind.

So we relax and re-teach, that is, "instruct" ourselves.

It is *not* the One-Day-At-A-Time Plan that causes you to lose all that poundage. It is *mainly* the new cause-effect subconscious learning that does it. And this is the way it should be.

John Doe does not overeat. He does not have false hunger or food cravings. He does not have any of your eating problems.

"Lucky John," you say. Maybe. However, John has other problems. He has unwanted cause-effect relationships, too. Maybe his body sweats profusely when he is anxious. Or maybe his head aches when he is tense.

Or maybe his gut aches when he is distraught.

Or maybe his skin itches when he is insecure.

Or maybe his hands shake when he is worried.

Or maybe he's tired when he is unhappy.

Or maybe his heart pounds when he feels guilty.

Or maybe he smokes incessantly, or drinks too much, or stutters, or has colds or ulcers when he is nervous or upset.

No one is totally free of unwanted mental "instructions." Poor John. Poor Mary. Poor until they replace these unwanted "instructions" with new ones.

Is this difficult to do? Not at all. It is so easy and effective that it is unbelievable. It was easy to learn to be the way we are. It will be just as easy to change this learning process.

You are relaxed as you read this book. You are learning about the wonderful changes that will happen to you. It has already begun to happen. New learning is beginning to be impressed in your subconscious mind.

Results:
 1. New behavior
 2. Uninterrupted, gratifying, easy weight loss

What You Have Every Right to Expect from the Schiff Plan

It happens so easily, almost automatically. Yet, *you* must participate. My patients cannot have someone attend my program for them. You cannot have someone read this book for you. You cannot lose weight by proxy. So here we are, you and I.

What happens next? What can you expect to happen as you read?

Remember I said this is a "total program." Reading is just part of it. Although reprogramming (replacing the old with new instructions) may already be underway for you, it may not yet be reflected on your scale. At present the reading is paving the way. Now it is providing general understanding about weight problems; later, specific understanding about yourself and your weight problem; still later, specific solutions for those problems.

The "total program" *is* the key. Food is one important aspect. But the mental aspect *is* the lock into which the key fits. This fit is accomplished one day at a time.

Place the key in the lock and the treasure chest opens! This treasure chest is so full of rewards that I am embarrassed to talk about them. Here is one of my patients describing the benefits she received 13 months into the total mind-body program. If the shoe fits, wear it. Otherwise, translate it into your own desires and life style:

"It's hard to put into words all the physical and mental changes that have occurred during the program. First the physical changes.

"I feel good. I feel more active . . . younger than I did a year ago. I'll be 41 next month. I feel more 'with it' than I did at 30. My daughters all say, 'Doesn't my mother look great at 40!'

"I have gone from a dress size 14 to a size 9. The inches lost are remarkable. Although I have lost relatively few pounds recently, I have continued to lose inches. I now have what I consider good proportions: chest 35, waist 25, hips 35.

"Another amazing physical change is the shape of my legs. On previous diets I lost weight, but never before in my kneecaps and in the width of my knees. I just bought several size 9, knee-length dresses. My family noticed the improvement in my legs. I was always concerned about my ugly knees and wore skirts that came below the knees. Now I have nice looking legs. At my age, this makes me very happy.

"The program has helped my mental and emotional condition. Without being self-centered or selfish, I have learned the importance of thinking and doing whatever is right for me. This has helped me to sort out the unimportant problems and events that used to 'bug' me.

"Also, I don't look too far ahead or feel uptight about my weight. I go, and do, one day at a time.

One day at a time. That's beautiful. It helped her to lose weight one pound at a time, from 155 to 120. And if you could weigh her thoughts, the scale would probably show considerable loss in the heavy, morose, down in the dumps department, as she became a happier, more confident, poised woman.

As you shed pounds off your body, you also shed excess baggage off your personality day by day.

Why You Don't Overeat and Regain in between Plan Days

If you went to a doctor's office for the purpose of losing weight, and he gave you a strict diet to follow for one month, what might happen?

Well, you would probably go home and eat your usual fare. "The doctor's menus start with breakfast. I'll begin tomorrow." The next morning you eat a diet breakfast "as prescribed." Your lunch, dinner, and snacks, too, are as the doctor ordered.

A few more days on the diet, maybe even a week or two, then something happens. Maybe a tray of desserts wheeled past you by a waiter. Or you go to a weekend party. Or your office cuts a cake to celebrate the Snodgrass contract. At any rate, you temporarily shelve the diet. One "sin" is followed by another, and it may be days or weeks later before you decide to "try again."

Let's examine what is really happening. You have been given instructions that do not conform with the way you have been behaving; eating incorrectly and overeating. It is, in effect, contradictory teaching. You now have two opposite sets of instructions in your mind. The result is conflict.

Whenever there is a conflict between two opponents, the stronger opponent prevails.

Which was the stronger teaching after the visit to the doctor? The old teaching by far. So, it prevailed or returned eventually. A victory for chocolate mousse, and hors d'oevre—ad infinitum.

You and I are *not* going on that trip.

First, there is no spelled-out diet, no counting calories and amounts of food.

Second, there is no spelled-out number of days, no time limits, no unreasonable, meaningless and self-defeating goals.

Instead of saying, at the end of one plan day, "I have to starve for 29 more days," you say, "well, that was easy enough. Do I have to quit? I'll repeat the One-Day-At-A-Time Plan tomorrow." And the probability is even greater that you'll say that and repeat it after the second day.

Even if you do not repeat the plan the very next day, a seed has been planted. That seed will grow. It is inevitable that one day soon you will remember the One Day, the good eating, the good feeling, the happy thoughts, the pound (or two or three) lost, and you will repeat it again.

Will you eat incorrectly the day after the plan day? Perhaps. But I am willing to bet that even if you decide not to repeat that One Day for weeks, your eating habits will improve because of the knowledge that you are receiving from these pages.

Already, you have a new concept of sugar and flour. Your menu is going to shift, subtly at first, then dramatically, away from foods with white sugar and white flour.

See for yourself. Do this experiment:

1. Record everything you eat today, from breakfast to dinner. Include drinks, snacks, even chewing gum. (There's white sugar going down your esophagus right now, if you are chewing gum.) Put down the estimated portion or weight in ounces.

2. One week from now, so it falls on the same day of the week, record your intake again in detail.

3. Using a standard calorie table, evaluate and compare the approximate decrease in white sugar and white flour calories for the weight of such foods eaten on both days.

Most women's magazines these days are a standoff. Half of the pages are devoted to fattening recipes, the other half to diets. The pages of the book you hold in your hand do not cancel each other out. They all add up. They all work for you. Meanwhile, your weight decreases.

Every page of this book is working for you. It is helping to program new insight, new nutrition, new confidence in setting and reaching your weight goal—one day at a time—one ounce at a time.

I think we are ready to take definitive steps in the program. Before you begin the next chapter, here are three things I want you to do:

1. Fill a container with water and place it in the refrigerator, if you do not already have one there. If you do, make sure it is full.

2. Obtain a notebook with at least a 5 x 9 page size, but larger is fine, and a sharpened pencil or ballpoint pen. Title the notebook "ME" and sign your name under it.

3. Find one or more items in your kitchen containing white sugar or made with white flour. Throw them in the garbage or give them to a neighbor or someone you don't like. Write down your feelings on page 2 of the notebook. What were your feelings as you gave or threw away the nonallowable items?

It has been nice meeting you. We are going to be close friends as we continue together. The *best* of friends.

III

ALL THE DELICIOUS FOOD YOU CAN EAT ON THE ONE-DAY-AT-A-TIME PLAN

Victor M., salesman, carried two notebooks wherever he went. One reminded him where to go and how to get there. It was his list of prospects for the day. The other was his One-Day notebook.

In this latter notebook, he recorded his eating and drinking; also his emotional ups and downs. "I lost the sale. Feeling disappointed and depressed, I stopped at Charlie's—had some pretzels and a few beers."

The prospect book mapped his business. The other book mapped his weight problem, certainly important business that was often sorely neglected. It provided him with a guide to the erroneous instructions which resulted in overeating and overdrinking.

The notebook you presumably now have will be an important part of the One-Day-At-A-Time concept.

No, you will not be eating it page by page. But even if you did, it would be a perfect, nonfattening snack as it consists of wood fiber, strictly bulk which your body would eliminate.

The importance of the notebook will be to guide you as well as to provide you with body and mind progress records day by day. *I repeat*, this notebook will be a valuable aid for you to initiate and to continue the One-Day-At-A-Time Plan.

The book you hold in your hands is my book. The notebook is your book. The two books complete a bridge between us, between "ME" (you) and me (Dr. Schiff).

Write "ME" on the cover. Underneath write "by" and your name. Now I would like you to prepare the table of contents on the first inside page. Number this page "1" in the upper right-hand corner.

Title this page at the top "Table of Contents." Copy the headings using the following diagram as a guide:

All the Delicious Food You Can Eat on the One-Day-At-A-Time Plan 45

ILLUSTRATION FOR A 50-PAGE NOTEBOOK

PAGE NO.	WEIGHT LOSS ACTIVITY	PROGRESS
2	Pre-Plan Sugar and Flour Intake	100%
3	New Sugar and Flour Intake	75%
4	Canceled Foods	50%
5	Allowable Foods	25%
6	Weight Record	
7	Measurement Record	
8	Health Record	
9-17	Meditations	
18-25	Self-Image	
26-33	Subconscious Instructions	
34 to End	Letters	

Now place the proper activity headings at the top of the correct pages as per your Table of Contents.

You are now ready to complete the third column, "Progress," located just to the right of each "Activity." Notice in the illustration how a line is drawn from left to right, giving you a ready visual indication of the extent of your progress. Executives find progress charts useful. So will you.

A short line means you have begun (25 percent). A line halfway across means you are halfway (50 percent) toward your goal. Keep working on each Activity until the lines extend all the way to the right-hand margin. This shows that you have completely (100 percent) accomplished that step (Activity).

Have you completed your record of today's sugar and flour intake (or yesterday's)? Then you can enter it on page 2 of your notebook—"Pre-Plan Sugar and Flour Intake Activity." Draw a thick line all the way across showing this step completed.

Later you can do the same for page 3, "New Sugar and Flour Intake Activity," thereby showing a reduced intake of those damaging sweets and starches. Again, make your thick record line on page 1, in the "Progress" column opposite "New Sugar and Flour Intake

Activity." Always record your progress by extending the record line toward the right margin by an amount that reflects the percentage of completion for each activity, that is, 25%, 50%, 75%, or 100%—see illustration on page 45.

I am going to discuss "Allowable Foods" with you. You will then be able to make suitable entries on page 5.

Here Is the Good News: This Is an Eating Program—Not a Noneating Program

Lamb chops, filet mignon, roast leg of veal.

This dish smothered in mushrooms. That dish sautéed with onions. Eat. Relax. Enjoy. Lose weight.

This is an eating program. We call it a One-Day-At-A-Time Plan, because we do change during that One Day, even though the physical and mental changes are not perceptible at the moment. The fare is so superb that it would be a mistake to call it a diet. It is a subtle shift rather than a strict diet. And the shift is to a world of wholesome, balanced, taste-tingling foods. It is a delicious shift. It is a one-day-at-a-time shift. It is a planned shift.

You *will not* begin your first day on the plan until you finish reading this book. If you wish to continue eating those doughnuts and danish, the pizza and the candy, until that day arrives, go ahead.

Meanwhile—here are the foods that are going to transform you into a more youthful, attractive, slender, and healthier person. (If you sense I am using some reverse psychology here, you are absolutely right.)

Basically, this is a high-protein, low-fat, low-carbohydrate weight-loss program.

High and low are relative terms. Measured a hundred years ago, no one would call this a low-fat, low-carbohydrate program. They would prefer to call it medium-fat, medium-carbohydrate—balanced, nutritious, enjoyable, slenderizing.

The reason is, we have unbalanced our food intake in the past century. We have become dairy rich (fats), and convenience oriented (carbohydrates).

So, basically, this is a balanced intake even though today it appears to be high in protein. And, even if it were imbalanced toward protein, our body prefers food angled in the protein direction. Given a say, the cells of our body would vote protein over fat and carbohydrate every time. I say, cast a "yes" vote for protein today.

Let's start with MEAT:

Allowed are all cuts of beef, veal and lamb. This includes round steak, pot roast, sirloin steak, rib roast, porterhouse steak, T-bone steak, rump steak, roast beef, chopped steak, flank steak, swiss steak, short ribs, beef liver, sweetbreads, kidney, brains. In the veal family are the same cuts and organs plus veal chops, both rib and loin. In the lamb family are also these cuts and organs plus leg of lamb. In the pork family, we run into high-fat meat. You can trim fat off beef and lamb—and when we talk about best ways to prepare meats we will emphasize the importance of trimming fat—but you cannot get the fat out of pork just by trimming. So choose pork chops only, trim, and cook well done.

Now POULTRY:

Allowed are all parts of the chicken—breast, thighs, legs, neck, wings. Avoid the skin, even if done to a crisp, as it is high in fat. Similarly, the turkey in all its glory is allowed. Lean to the white meat; it's leaner than the dark. Squab, pheasant, cornish hen, and other game birds are fine but make a wide circle around duck or goose—too much fat. Most Americans seldom eat duck and have never tasted goose, so you probably are not being deprived in this department.

FISH AND SEAFOOD:

Cultivate a taste for fish—it's a great protein food. All fish are allowable. To name just a few—tuna, salmon, cod, halibut, flounder, bass, trout, haddock, sturgeon, whitefish, finnan haddie, perch, herring, red snapper, mackerel, sole, abalone, anchovy, pickerel, shad, bonito, eel, barracuda, marlin. Prefer fresh and frozen fish to salted, pickled, and smoked. Seafood (shellfish) varieties allowed are again total—crab, clam, lobster, oyster, mussel, shrimp, scallop, crayfish, and snail. Canned, minced, smoked, etc. are less desirable protein than fresh and frozen. Avoid fried fish and seafood that has been coated with bread crumbs for frying; avoid fish cakes as they're stuffed with cereal filling.

CHEESE:
There is more good eating here and good protein. Investigate new cheeses but be aware of fat content. Cheese specialty stores can suggest variety and advise about fat content. Lean toward the low-fat cheeses. Here are some—American, Camembert, Cheddar, Cottage, Edam, Farmers, Gouda, Gruyere, Mozzarella, Muenster, Parmesan, Pot, Provolone, Ricotta, Romano, Swiss, and Tilsiter. Avoid high-fat cheeses, such as Cream Cheese. Treat cheese with reverence; savor every morsel. Snack all you want on Pot Cheese and Farmers Cheese.

VEGETABLES:
Above ground, leafy kinds are best. Preferred, above or below ground, are asparagus, beet greens, broccoli, cabbage, carrots, cauliflower, celery, chard, chicory, Chinese cabbage, collard greens, cucumber, dandelion greens, endive, escarole, kale, kohlrabi, leek, mushroom, mustard greens, onions, peppers, dill pickles, pimentos, radishes, rhubarb, scallions, spinach, squash (zucchini), string beans, turnip, watercress. Tomatoes (actually a fruit) are acceptable.

SALAD:
Many of the above vegetables, raw, make excellent salad material, such as spinach leaves, shredded cabbage, cucumber slices, onions, peppers, and scallions. Also acceptable—tomatoes. Then, of course, there are the many varieties of lettuce, for the body of your salad plus the leaves of the celery, onion grass, and add a sprig of parsley. Use low-calorie (diet) dressing only. This is lower in oil content, and no sugar has been added. Or make your own dressing: one part safflower oil, three parts vinegar. Use sparingly.

EGGS:
Boiled, baked, scrambled, fried, souflèed, and in omelets. Any style, but don't use butter or oil. Instead, cook on a Teflon-coated pan or any pan that does not require fat or oil, or use Panstick, Pam, Teflon Spray, etc.

FRUIT *(Once a Day)*:
Preferred fruits are grapefruit (½); cantaloupe, honeydew, casaba, and watermelon; strawberries, blackberries, and gooseberries; peaches, pears, and plums. All fruit portions should be small and, since fruit is

high in carbohydrate, eat it only once a day. Fresh fruit is preferred. If frozen, avoid sugar-added types. If canned, avoid the syrup pack—use the natural juice pack. Slice the fruit in half or into thirds to make it last longer.

BEVERAGES:
The more water the better. Drink at least four or five glasses of water a day and at least eight glasses total of liquid a day. Other liquids allowed include tea—weak is preferred, adding lemon is permitted—and coffee, decaffeinated only, and black. Coffee lovers should make this switch to decaffeinated as it reduces nervousness, provides less gastric stimulation, and cuts up-and-down blood sugar cycles that create false hunger; a couple of glasses of buttermilk or non-fat milk are allowed; low-calorie soft drinks, three or less calories per can, are allowed, but keep your drinking down to two cans a day as the chemicals that are used as sugar substitutes are a problem to some people. Later, I will give you recipes for special drinks that I "concocted" for my own as well as my patients' health and pleasure—such as my Protein Punch and my Energy Sling—drinks that quench not only thirst but hunger as well.

QUANTITY:
Eat all you need to satisfy true hunger. If weight reaches a plateau, first decrease fruit intake, followed by a decrease of vegetables. Be sure the remaining fruits and vegetables are the lowest calorie varieties. Proteins should be those with the least fat content.

There you have it. It is tough in areas of indulgence, but it is permissive in areas of protein-rich nutrition. It provides a no-nonsense, balanced food intake that will produce results in One Day.

That One Day will make you so enthusiastic about the eating enjoyment-weight loss combination that you will want to repeat it again and again.

It will be just exactly the opposite of the 10-day, 20-day, or 30-day diets where you counted the days and maybe you lasted and maybe you didn't. Instead, you won't be able to wait to go back on that enjoyable One-Day Plan.

Now copy into your notebook (page 5) from the above lists of allowable foods all those you enjoy and are familiar with, plus any you would like to sample. This becomes your shopping and menu-planning guide.

Selections, One Day At A Time

The choice of *if* or *when* you continue the plan for another day is strictly yours to make.

You continue the plan one day at a time. You do not push yourself. You can repeat the One-Day Plan again next week or next month or next year. You can go on it again tomorrow, or never.

If you go on it again tomorrow, it is because you gain in eating pleasure, in vigor, in energy, and in joie de vivre as you drop those few ounces or few pounds. You enjoy and accept whatever happens. You make a beautiful happening. You make *it* happen.

If you never repeat it again, it is quite likely because it has made its mark on you and you are no longer in need of it, that is you recognize false hunger (appetite) by using the instructions and "how to" directions on the pages ahead and you defuse false instructions in ways I will point out. You have shifted by pure common sense away from sickly sweet and starchy foods to the foods that keep you alive and well. And you have shifted from a negative to a positive polarity, from failure to success, from joyless to joyful.

What a difference this recognition, defusing, and shifting will make in your weight over the months ahead, and in your peace of mind and health of body, all from that one day!

Later, I will give you "switch plans" to make each repeat a gratifying and meaningful adventure. These will include a protein-supplemental plan using the predigested protein drink (only one daily); a portion-cutting plan; and others. The basic theory is to keep yourself happy and having fun as you lose weight. You have so many ways to construct your selections for one day that you will probably want to make your own variations day to day.

There is a large span between restrictiveness versus permissiveness, between plain versus gourmet, between one taste preference versus a completely different taste preference. For instance, here are two One-Day selections, the one on the left recorded by Violet F., the one on the right by Fred L.

All the Delicious Food You Can Eat on the One-Day-At-A-Time Plan 51

Violet F.	Fred L.
7:00 a.m.—½ cup cottage cheese black coffee	6:30 a.m.—two fried eggs one veal kidney coffee, black
10:30 a.m.—½ grapefruit 1 hard-boiled egg black coffee	12:00 p.m.—3 oz. hamburger steak cole slaw coffee, black bread, 1 slice
12:30 p.m.—tomato cheese omelet green salad black coffee	3:00 p.m.—1 oz. cheese slices diet soda
3:30 p.m.—black coffee	
6:30 p.m.—3 oz. broiled chicken 2 fresh mushrooms 2 oz. gouda cheese black coffee	7:00 p.m.—2 veal chops bread, ½ slice asparagus mixed green salad honeydew melon coffee, black
8:30 p.m.—diet soda	

The left-hand diet is "rigid." The right-hand plan is "loose."

Which results in the most weight loss?

Well, the rigid diet may eliminate 2½ pounds, depending on weight, activities, metabolism, and chemistry of the person making the decision and selection. However, the loss may not be repeated. You may not enjoy the rigidity and decide not to duplicate that diet day again.

On the other hand, the "loose plan" may remove only a fraction of an ounce or pound during that one day. However, the weight loss may continue if one chooses to repeat the "loose plan" every second day, or third day, or once a week—one day at a time. Within a few weeks or a month the "loose plan" could result in more weight loss than the "rigid" diet.

You make the decision. Florence E. made the selection and the decision to repeat. She was shy and retiring when I first met the 194 pounds of her. Little wonder—a 16-year-old girl with all that fat is embarrassed more than an adult who has adjusted somewhat to the problem.

After the first day, Florence wrote, "I didn't actually feel I was on a diet. The feeling of being on a diet is really like a hell to me. It turns me off like crazy. Like for me at age 16, going out to lunch with friends and on weekends can be boring on a diet. This, though, is not a diet, just a change, a new way of eating, thinking, and doing. It becomes a challenge. It makes life better for me, my body and mind. It is exciting, not boring."

Florence repeated the selections frequently because she enjoyed the challenge and the excitement of a more socially acceptable teenager emerging from that mound of fat.

In 12 weeks she lost 34 pounds—and was still counting down. "I am more important to me than all the bread I used to eat. The strange thing is I don't miss it at all. I have finally found a job. They picked me because of my outgoing personality. Can you believe that shy me, now outgoing! I feel so happy. I feel like a new person. I can hardly believe this is me. It's amazing! It's almost like a miracle!"

This is Florence's food intake her first day on the Plan—her menu for the correct and enjoyable eating day. Alongside is her menu for a diet day. Can you tell which was her diet day intake and which is now her correct eating day intake? Incidentally, Florence is not a breakfast eater, so no breakfasts appear on either day.

	Diet day or correct eating day?	*Diet day or correct eating day?*
Lunch	hamburger with one piece of bread; soda	beef stew; cheese; mixed green salad; coffee, black
Early afternoon snack:	fish sandwich with one piece of bread; soda	fish slices; soda
Dinner:	chicken and rice	chicken, vegetables, skim milk

Snack: vanilla wafers, milk   pear, black coffee

Answer: the right-hand column is Florence's food intake on her first correct eating day—her version of the One-Day-At-A-Time Plan. On the left is the food she used to eat on a typical diet day. There is something I didn't mention as it would give away the answer. The soda she drank on the correct eating day, the day of improved food intake, was diet (low-calorie) soda. The diet days she drank coke (high-calorie).

You may find that after being on the Plan for only one day, as you grow leaner, subsequent diet days will lean in the direction of the correct eating (Plan) days. Not because you have to. Because you *want* to. And—because you *do*.

You will not have to decide now. You will not have to decide when you are through reading this book and are ready to begin. You may never have to make the decision of how many times, if any, you will repeat the correct eating (Plan) day. Just "hang loose."

Enjoy yourself. Enjoy eating and losing weight—just one day at a time.

Yesterday, Today, and Tomorrow

Can you enjoy eating while you are in physical pain? Hardly. Can you enjoy eating while you are in mental pain? Same answer. Aristotle said learning is accompanied by pain. Publilius Syrus agreed when he said that the pain of the mind is worse than the pain of the body.

We can take an aspirin for a headache. But if we have a heartache, we usually take food as a pain reliever. We eat to forget our mental torment, our loneliness, our insecurity, our disturbed thoughts and distressed feelings, and so on.

There is an antidote.

That antidote for mental torment is: *Live well today*.

I say to you now—and don't go on to the next page until you think about and understand what I am saying—*look to this day only*.

If you live in a world of yesterdays, you are living in a dream world, and some of the dreams are nightmares.

If you live in a world of tomorrows, you are living in a world of visions, most of them fantasies.

However, if you live in a world of todays, living well today, then all of your yesterdays become accomplishments and all of your tomorrows become ambitions to be realized.

Are you drowning in a bowl of self-pity? Are you stifling in a platter of remorse? Are you decaying in a dish of self-negation? Then climb out now. Don't lose another day of the happiness that life has in store for you—that you have stored within *you*.

Decide now—to live the way you want to live. Do, say, think, and be. If you do not do, you will instead eat. If you do not say, you will instead stuff food into your mouth. If you do not think, you will instead munch. If you do not agree to be yourself, you will continue to be the overweight person who you know is not the real you.

In April, 1977, Donna Y. came to my office. I looked at her. Why was an old woman dressed so slovenly? Then I looked at the report filled out by my nurse. Donna was only 51. She was dressed in a dirty sweatshirt and sloppy pants. She weighed 171. She said she wanted to lose 35 pounds.

Donna wore no make-up. Her hair was a mess. She needed a bath. Her appearance belied her 51 years.

I decided I would convince Donna to talk about herself, and this is what emerged: She had a terrible craving for sweets all the time. Yes, she always dressed that way. Why? "I don't think about myself. I think about and do for others." She said she always thought about others first. She never considered her own needs.

"Why do you want to lose weight?" I asked. "To make my husband happy," was her reply.

Donna went ahead with the weight-control program.

The program requires that you place yourself ahead of others. This is not selfish love. It is instead *self-love*—to think, understand, enjoy, accept, learn about, and do for yourself. For Donna, it was a complete about-face. Her attitude about herself had to change. And when it did, her weight did an about-face, too.

Within three months, she lost 25 of those 35 pounds. She was grooming her hair, using some eye shadow and lipstick, and wearing stylish clothes. Now, she looked much younger than her years. She admitted that men were complimenting her and women were less friendly.

"What about your craving for sweets?" I asked.

She replied with one word: "Yuk."

"Me" had taken the place of "meal." The meals she had made of chocolates and ice cream sundaes were replaced by sweetness to herself, nonfattening sweetness. Before, she had developed a problem with her hurting feet. Now they were fine. Before, she felt it an effort to do her office work and was making mistakes. Now her brain seemed to have "come alive."

"The most important thing in my life now is *me*," she said emphatically.

"What about your husband?" I asked, remembering that he too had suffered because of her former problem.

"Would you like to meet him? He's in the reception room."

He was a tall, athletic man about 60. He told me what a great change had taken place in his wife and how this program also made him feel young again. He had changed his eating habits, too; he felt more energetic and was now playing volleyball. He showed me a sprained finger to prove it.

I see so many Donnas—women who have decided they are nobody. Today is not for them. They have no life today. They take part in other people's lives, but not their own.

Take Sharon. Her face was wrinkled. At 153 she was nearly 30 pounds overweight. At 59, she looked 69. Soon after beginning the One-Day-At-A-Time Plan, with her weight descending, she decided to have a face peel. This is a process that removes wrinkles. What a breakthrough. Sharon was deciding to live her own life again.

A year later, Sharon's wrinkles were gone, she was a slender 125. "After years of hating myself," she said, "I'm excited and delighted about myself. Thinking and doing on a daily basis was the clincher."

It happens with men, too. Al S. was really a big one. Not vertically. Horizontally. He weighed 245. He was only 35 years old, but he dressed sloppily and went unshaven. Needless to say, his work as a home improvement salesman suffered. Who would buy from someone who lived in a "home" like his and looked like him?

Al kept to himself when he wasn't at work. He had no desire to do anything, no energy. He had little to say to anyone. Let's face it, he didn't have much of a life of his own.

How fortunate that people such as Al decide to make a change. When they come to my office, they have already made a decision to reclaim their lives—to live once again for today. Otherwise I would never see them.

You, *too*, have made a decision or you would not be reading this book. I am delighted for you, too. And I feel the importance of my responsibility to you, no less than to my office patients, to help you live *your* life fully again.

Well, Al did just that. As he began to "open up" mentally, his body closed up physically. As Al became more interested in himself, he became less interested in gorging food and processed junk. He shaved every day and dressed smartly. He lost 62 pounds in four months, was given a promotion on his job, and went on camping trips again with new friends.

He lived each day, fully. He lived and achieved one day at a time.

You need to start by living well today, just for you. *You* are the most important person in your life. This is *your* life, only. Make yourself the most beautiful and important person you possibly can. And believe my countless, successful, slender patients—you can!

Say Goodbye to Your Old Self

Have you entered the allowable foods into your book? If not, please do so now.

I am going to list the nonallowable foods now, but I want to make sure you examine them against a backdrop of the great eating and abundant gustatory pleasure you derive from the allowable foods.

These nonallowable foods are the sweets, starches, and fats. Some of them are obvious. Others are more secretive about their fat and carbohydrate content.

Look at the nonallowable foods listed below as the old you. You are discarding these foods. And in the process, you are discarding the old you day by day. This permits the new you to emerge and enjoy life, one great day at a time.

MEAT:
No ham or pork (except lean pork chops, well done). No bacon. No hot dogs, or smoked meats. No sausage, bologna, or similar "cold cuts."

POULTRY:
No duck or goose.

FISH:
Avoid smoked fish and sardines.

CHEESE:
No cream cheese. Avoid soft cheese. Usually light yellow cheese contains less fat than dark yellow cheese.

VEGETABLES:
No potatoes or potato chips, no corn or popcorn, no rice or cornstarch, no starchy vegetables, such as peas, lima beans, and sweet potatoes.

SALAD:
No salad dressings except low-calorie preparations (read the labels carefully), or your own mixture of safflower oil and vinegar.

FRUIT:
No avocados, bananas, cherries, dates. No dried fruits. No fruits canned in syrup. No apple or orange juice. On occasion, only a few grapes, an orange or apple wedge—but check the pointer on the scale carefully. Remember, fruits that are allowed should be limited to one portion per day.

DAIRY:
No milk, whole or evaporated (except buttermilk or skimmed milk or non-fat powdered); no butter, cream, margarine, mayonnaise, or flavored yogurt. Occasionally, a small amount of low-fat, plain yogurt is permissible.

GRAINS:
No baked goods such as cakes, biscuits, crackers, pancakes, waffles, pies. Bread (freshly milled, stone ground)—1 or 2 slices daily depending on progress. If indicated, eliminate for a while. No cereals, hot or cold. No cookies, doughnuts, pastry. No pretzels or rolls. No spaghetti and other pastas.

BEVERAGES:

No coffee except decaffeinated. No tea, except weak, decaffeinated, or herbal. No soda except diet soda (3 calories or less per can). No alcoholic beverages.

DESSERTS:

No candy, no ice cream or ices, no sweet toppings. No nuts, seeds, coconut. No chocolate or cocoa. No jams, jellies, preserves, marmalade, or honey.

These foods belong to the old you. The old you belongs to the past. The past changes to the new future with the one day of correct and enjoyable eating—one day at a time.

A *new you is born*. Happy Birthday!

Do Not Begin the One-Day-At-A-Time Plan Yet Because . . .

You now know what to eat and what not to eat on that One Day. Copy the nonallowable foods into the proper page (No. 4) of your book entitled "ME." You will note there are fewer nonallowable, and more allowable.

Once entries are completed on both pages 4 and 5, mark the progress lines accordingly on your contents page (No. 1). Bring the bar lines all the way over to the right side of the page, showing at a glance that this part has been completed.

The One-Day-At-A-Time Plan is not to be started now. Patience. It is not to begin until all the progress bar lines extend over to the edge or right-hand margin, showing completion of these prerequisites. It is not to begin until you have finished reading this book. Why? Otherwise it will be just another diet instead of a total program. Reading this book, then using the "How to" directions and instructions, is an important part of the program.

Today, people realize that body, mind, and spirit all need to be healthy for total health. This means a "Holistic" program, a program devoted to you—the complete you.

Here is what to expect in the pages ahead.

I want you to know how best to prepare different foods. I want you to know all about soups, gravies, and spices.

I want you to know how to derive the most nourishment from the mere enjoyment of food and from the least number of calories.

You will learn how to add more meals to the day to help you actually lose weight and become slender.

Did you know there are ways to handle your knife and fork to make a meal seem larger and last longer? You are going to learn these "tricks." They help to increase your eating enjoyment without increasing your weight.

You are going to learn how to differentiate between *appetite* and *hunger. Appetite is emotional and psychological.* You can suppress true hunger with a pill, but there is no pill that will suppress appetite because it is false hunger.

So, you will *learn to feed your hunger* and feed it well. But you will *learn to cope with your appetite (emotions, feelings)* in a different way, so that appetite will no longer masquerade as the need for food.

You are going to learn to take care of yourself. You are going to treat yourself better than anyone has ever treated you. You are going to pamper yourself. You are going to learn to know yourself better. And you are going to love this person, "ME." As you learn to take care of yourself, the weight will take care of itself. And the pointer on the scale will move downward day by day.

You are going to see the funny side of life. You are going to see that many of your problems are actually other people's problems. It will tickle you in the ribs, and your ribs will become more accessible to be tickled.

You are going to acquire a new feeling about yourself. You are going to have a new appearance. Even without beginning the One-Day-At-A-Time Plan, you will stand taller, appear younger, look more radiant and alive as your outward appearance reflects a more confident, peaceful inner self.

There is more.

I will want you to exercise your body. A moderate amount is desirable, and I will show you how this can do the most good. We will be using exercise in a different way. Not to burn off calories. That requires long stretches of strenuous, boring work. Forget it. We will do it the easy way—using exercise as a mental aid: tension easer, psychic relaxer, boredom breaker, emotional releaser, and eating-urge interrupter. Secondary physical benefits of these exercises will be as limber uppers, slimmer downers, calorie expenders, muscle toners and beautifiers, to help your body regain its youthful expression and slender contour.

I will want you to exercise and beautify your mind (have beautiful thoughts). I will teach you in the pages ahead an easy way to write about yourself that will release pounds of fat. Yes, there are mental factors that the pounds "hang" on to. Eliminate these and the fat falls off, swiftly.

You begin to recognize these factors as you write in the book called "ME." Once recognized, you automatically detour around them. You handle them. Unknown, they form roadblocks that handle you. Don't mishandle yourself.

I will teach you to reprogram your mental "computer" (self-instruct) so you'll think, eat, and behave as a slender person.

I will help you *to understand* and *to love yourself*—one day at a time. You'll find there is no one quite like you in this whole world, that you are indeed a unique and attractive individual, that today is really the first day of the rest of your life—a now exciting life for a new alluring you.

IV

GROUND RULES FOR THE ONE-DAY-AT-A-TIME PLAN

Oscar C. went on the One-Day-At-A-Time Plan and lost 52 pounds in 112 days.

Marion R. went on the One-Day-At-A-Time-Plan and lost 12 pounds in 115 days.

Both were successful.

The reason for this big difference in amount of weight loss: for Oscar time was important, whereas Marion knew she was going to be slender a long time. A few months or more of waiting to enjoy her new life style mattered less than the ultimate attainment of her slender goal.

Oscar went one day at a time for 112 successive days.

Marion went one day at a time just five or six times in a 115-day span.

How fast or slowly you wish to lose weight is your decision. I set a number of ground rules for you on the Plan, but losing a pound a week or three pounds a week is not one of them. Don't set yourself up for a letdown with unrealistic goals and self-defeating expectations.

I will give you a number of ways to accelerate your weight loss if time is important to you. Repeating the One Day more frequently is one of them. But you are going to be adding many healthy, happy, attractive, slender years to your life. So don't sweat. Relax. Take it easy. Enjoy.

I don't want you to waste any effort in this final slenderizing of yourself. I want you to lose unwanted bulges efficiently, effortlessly, and effectively.

If you have to use willpower, if you have to try, you are just buying yourself an undesirable, new lease on fat-dom. I want the plan to be sheer eating pleasure and joyous thinking so you can coast through each "one day" as easy as pie.

And that is the first important ground rule.

Ground Rule Number One—No Willpower, No Trying

If it takes willpower not to eat something that is "off limits" for the One Day, I'd rather you eat it and move on to another day. It is easier to do something. It requires more effort not to do something. For the present, limit those "No-No's" and cut portions in half. Later, I will give you methods for directing the mind to dislike chocolate cake or jelly beans or any other fattening food.

Meanwhile, develop the capacity to substitute for both fattening and junk foods.

I will be giving you methods for directing the mind if those fattening and junk foods continue to confront you. But under *no* conditions do I want you to "try."

Do you know why I am so lenient? It is not leniency. It is common sense. If you can't beat 'em, join 'em. And you can't beat a sweet or other irresistible foods with willpower or by trying. It takes some other method.

Ground Rule Number One is "Do not try. Don't use willpower."

Do what you want to do. Eat what you want to eat. Either remain on the Plan that day or delay it to another day. But do remember that repeated delays may dissipate your desire and capacity to achieve your ultimate goal.

By not trying and gradually easing into the One-Day-At-A-Time Plan, you tap the power of the normally slender person who does not "try" either. As a bonus, you develop the capacity to eat and think correctly—and to shed excess pounds day by day.

Then you become that normally slender person yourself.

Don't Count Calories, Count "Kiks"

This is an eating program, not a noneating program.

In a noneating program, you limit your intake of food by counting calories. You limit your total food for the day to 1200 calories or 800 calories or 1500 calories, depending on, if you will pardon my cynicism, how soon you want to fail.

In an eating program there is no counting calories. Instead, you keep track of your enjoyment. The more enjoyment, the sooner and more assured you are of success.

How do you measure enjoyment? Well, if you get a kick out of Beef Stroganoff, just how much kick did you get? I say, measure enjoyment by "kicks," and I call that unit of enjoyment the "kik." In this program you don't count calories, you count "kiks." The "kik" is not based on amount of food; it is based on deliciousness. It is qualitative, not quantitative. More "kiks" equals more food enjoyment, more personal enjoyment—and less weight.

So we *do not* limit enjoyment as the calorie system does. We strive for greater enjoyment, for more "kiks." In this program life can become abundantly filled with "kiks."

You can make a self-rating system. How much did you enjoy your breakfast today, say on a scale of 1-10? Also, rate your lunch, dinner, and snacks on a scale of 1-10. Then when you start this program, rate your enjoyment of that one day. It must equal or exceed previous scores. If it doesn't, then add some enjoyable foods from your "allowable list" so that your score will go up. It will help your weight go down.

Disallowed foods are not enjoyable because they represent failure and are fattening. And that's definitely no fun—it's downright "kikless."

Allowed foods are eligible to be enjoyed, but people have different tastes. You need to pick the allowable foods that give you more "kiks." And prepare them so you'll derive maximum enjoyment.

Calorie counting and anxiety about calories means less enjoyment, more hardship, greater willpower, trying harder, eventual failure. More "kiks" means more enjoyment, no hardship, no willpower, greater ease, eventual success.

Do you see why this is a gratifying plan? It is gratifying the first day because it means changing. But the change is to greater enjoyment, not less. So the change sticks, and the pounds leave—swiftly.

Look for more ways of eating enjoyment with allowable foods. Plan your menus for fun. Cook the food for fun. Cook with you in mind.

Eat allowable snacks for fun. Eat for "kiks." *Eat to enjoy.*

This is Ground Rule number two.

Substitute Quality for Quantity

Your body is *your* responsibility. Nobody is going to feed or take care of it for you.

The body does not thrive on carbohydrates. It does not thrive on fat. It thrives on protein, minerals, and vitamins. It can utilize a little oil and some fibers or roughage.

But if your body were to make known its own enjoyment to you measured by nutritional "kiks," it would flash on the "kik" sign for meat, poultry, and fish, for low-fat cheese, for raw leafy greens and vegetables, and that raw apple, peach, or pear.

Your body would flash on the "foul" sign for sweets, starches, and fats; for prepared foods that have more chemicals, colorants, and preservatives than nutrients; for foods that are overcooked, with nutrients burned or dissolved out.

You feed your face, but starve your body, when you eat these foods. Net result: You hunger quickly and need to eat more; you need extra "kiks." But it is usually false hunger (appetite).

When you substitute quality for quantity, your enjoyment goes up as your quantity goes down.

Ground Rule number three: cut your portions in half as you double your nutrition.

On the pages ahead I will be helping you to recognize the best foods and how to cook them to retain their goodness and their nutrition.

Half-sized portions eaten leisurely and enjoyed forkful by forkful are twice as large as full portions wolfed down.

When you are aware of a portion of filet of fish, discontinue conversation or stop your thoughts from roaming as the fork enters your mouth. By experiencing the taste of the fish, each mouthful does double duty for you in eating satisfaction; thus, you are satisfied with half as much.

Your body has less digestive work to do for greater nutrition. Your nerves are steadier. You are more composed. You are better able to cope with life's problems. As stress is less, your health improves. And your fun in life improves as your weight descends.

Sheila U., 43, and a teacher, weighed 216, about 70 pounds more than she should. She enjoyed the Weight-Control Plan so much she stayed on it 15 months. During this time her weight dropped slowly but surely, week after week, month after month. She had no sense of dieting, no counting calories, no striving to last out another week or month. She stayed on allowed foods and half portions because it made for good eating, but it also brought other changes for Sheila.

She had always been in a hurry, nervous, unhappy, and beset by marital difficulties. Her husband depended upon her for support and did nothing around the house. She conveyed her annoyance with him to her students. In order to ease her annoyance, she stuffed herself with food.

As she embarked on the program and found herself extending it one day at a time, her nerves gradually calmed down. She had a feeling of well-being which she brought into her classroom. The students responded with better attention and behavior, and her job became easier and more enjoyable. She decided to see a psychiatrist about her marital problem (her husband refused any therapy) and developed enough inner strength to divorce him, "which I should have done years ago." Sheila U. is now a slender, successful teacher, and a happy person. Sheila U. is now Sheila G., weight 144 pounds.

You will discover benefits in your own life that will accumulate as unexpected dividends in addition to your weight loss. They will be mental as well as physical. As you lose a piece of your body, called fat, you gain peace of mind—one day at a time.

Ground Rule Number Four—The Startling "Rule of Two."

Get ready for a surprise. I want you to eat two more meals every day. If you eat three meals a day, I want you to eat five meals a day. If you eat two meals a day, I want you to eat four meals a day. Even if you are now eating four meals a day, please make it six—six mini-meals.

Cancel the word "please." *I insist.*

In fact, adding two more mini-meals every single day is Ground Rule number four. You have no option. It is required.

All four Ground Rules contribute to your hearty enjoyment of food. Ground Rule One = no willpower or trying. Ground Rule Two = tastier food (more "kiks"). Ground Rule Three = more nourishing food, yet less quantity. Ground Rule Four = more daily occasions to apply rules one, two, and three by using the "Rule of Two."

Why more meals? To keep your stomach full. To keep your mind at ease. And, to keep your body at ease.

If you skip meals, as most diets encourage you to do by their calorie-conscious approach, you will fail.

If you add meals, and avoid any periods of false hunger, you will increase and consolidate your feeling of pleasure and ease—and you will succeed.

You can add the two meals whenever you wish. However, the total quantity of food each day is important and must be gradually decreased whenever the pointer on the scale pauses for a prolonged period of time. You'll find it takes no willpower to reduce portions when you add meals (mini-meals).

You can have a second breakfast, or a late afternoon tea, or a midnight snack.

If you are currently skipping breakfast, I recommend you add a meal here.

But the choice is yours. Just remember that the plan has hundreds of allowable foods, a lifetime of satisfying, even gourmet dining. There is no need to deviate for enjoyment's sake, or for hunger's sake or, for the sake of mental ease. You can feel secure that all your past eating pleasure is safe in the future on this program. You will discover this yourself when you go on it for one day.

No doctor can force a patient to "stick to a diet." That is why bariatrics (weight control) is a frustrating practice for many physicians who choose this branch of medicine.

"Try it—for one day." What patient can refuse that request, especially when the pains and problems of obesity are compared to the benefits and blessings of an attractive silhouette.

So you go on it for one day.

Now, when you do something different and it is not enjoyable, you are not likely to choose to do it again. You may have to a few times, or you may push yourself to do it again, but eventually you quit—"I've had it!"

So you go off it indefinitely. And the weight returns.

But when you do something different and it is enjoyable, you choose it again and again. And you do it again and again.

So it is one day at a time. And so it was with Carole E.

Ground Rules for the One-Day-At-A-Time Plan 67

You would not believe how Carole looked at 35. She weighed only 154, which for her frame and height was really only 20 percent overweight. But on her it hung, it clouded, and it uglified.

She seemed to reflect in her face her lack of interest about her appearance and a sort of hopelessness—such as using no make-up, permitting dark facial hair to dominate her upper lip and chin, and wearing a hair style perfect for someone who owned no comb or brush.

Carole told me about her health problems. She had frequent headaches and was plagued with asthma. She was taking injections for the asthma and pills for the headaches. She wished there was a pill that would make her two teenage daughters behave and also ease the constant bickering and hostility in the family.

"I've never been able to stay on a diet, doctor," she warned me. "Diet pills would be better."

"Go on this program for just one day." I replied, "It is different."

I gave her the list of allowable foods and explained about the quality of food ("kiks") and the "Rule of Two," and so on.

Carole started the program and liked it. She stayed on it, with very few days as exceptions. In seven months her weight dropped from 154 to 123. By then, consciously, she paid scant attention to what she was eating—her understanding about herself, about foods and the ability to control food intake, was now automatic. She continued to lose weight and within two months dropped another nine pounds.

She looked younger and the sags and bulges that previously blurred her features were gone. Here now was an alive, radiant face. She bleached her dark facial hair. She used a touch of make-up. She styled her hair. She went from hag to chick.

But that was only half the story. As she lost weight her health improved. The headaches disappeared. She was able to handle the asthma without injections. Her nerves were steady. She felt more energetic and became more effective. Although the daughters were still involved with their own problems, they no longer created family tension. Life for Carole had improved immeasurably. Carole had improved herself immeasurably.

And it all happened one day—a day so structured that it led to another, and another—and another.

Now for Ground Rule Five.

How to Act Like a Slender Person and Hasten That Day

Our thoughts control our behavior. We think about doing something and we do it.—Or, we don't do it.

A man who thinks about being a big executive acts like one and begins to become one. A young man who thinks mostly of "making it" with girls acts and looks quite differently than a young man who thinks primarily of furthering his academic career. And the same is true of a young girl who thinks more about boys than books and knowledge. We begin to look and act like the person we think we are.

The overweight person who accepts the chubby picture, acts like a chubby person, and certainly looks like one. The overweight person who sees (visualizes) instead the slender person that he or she actually is inside, does not appear to be as heavy as the scale somberly declares. His or her body "language" is different. They walk with a lighter step despite the excess weight. The movements of the body are more graceful and lithe despite the cumbersome dimensions.

When you think thin, you hasten the day.

But you have to mean it, then *do* something about it each day.

You have to plan for the day when you become a thin person. For example, you may take an interest in clothing styles that are not right for you today, but will be right for you one day. Go to a store and actually select what you will one day wear. Don't purchase it yet, but make a mental note to purchase it later.

Stand erect. Hold your body in a more slender posture, even if it requires muscle power. Get the body started in the slender direction by having it follow your slender (positive) thinking.

Begin to act as though you were the center of attraction. Male or female, look your best. Acquire the habit of being meticulously dressed. Be proud of your appearance.

Now, I'm not saying that such thoughts, and the actions to suit them, will make you thin. But they will definitely help.

Weight will burn off your body faster if your mind is helping the body in that direction. *The pathway to your body is through your mind.* Your mind controls your body. Instruct your mind to control.

A fat, lazy, slovenly, pessimistic outlook begets a body to fit that outlook. It will indeed become an imperfect fit.

Ground Rule number five is: Think thin, act thin, do thin, be thin. And, eat correctly to be and to stay thin. You can begin practicing this Ground Rule now.

An excellent way is to take a daily walk. Don't use a walk to the market or to the office for this purpose. Take those walks also. But take an extra walk daily. It need only be a few minutes. Start the day or end the day with a special, brisk walk. A walk for walking's sake.

Carry nothing with you. Swing your arms. Feel the spring in your step. Imagine that you are smaller around the hips. Pretend that you are slender as you walk. Get the "feel" of being slender. Know that you'll soon be slender.

The special daily walk is one way you can make the slender image of yourself a daily habit. The thoughts you have of yourself while walking will tend to repeat themselves during the day as you move from here to there. You will be instructing your body to slim down to its proper size. Eventually the body will respond.

An Unexpected Daily Source of Fat

Ground Rule Number Six is going to surprise you.

Remember, we talked about the mind's role in running the body? We are using that fact in Ground Rule Number Five—setting up a mental climate of slenderness as we walk and move about.

But it goes beyond that. You can actually reduce your caloric intake by foregoing certain thoughts. You are hearing me correctly. Do without certain erroneous thoughts and you do without certain excessive calories.

Let me explain. You and I have emotions (feelings). You may deal with your emotions one way, and I may deal with my emotions another way. I might become bored and decide to go on a weekend trip. You might become bored and decide to take a trip too—to the refrigerator. I may become angry and use the telephone to straighten someone out. You may become angry and go on an eating binge.

I might become lonesome if my family is away and go see a movie, visit a friend, or read a book. You might become lonesome and go to a restaurant or a bar, or raid the refrigerator. I am slender. You are overweight.

We all learned or were instructed how to use food as a soothing device in infancy. The baby who cries for love and attention is fed. Food becomes a substitute for love. If love is not around, there is always some lovely food around.

Parents reinforce this as the child grows older. If a child behaves well, candy or dessert is offered as a reward. If a child is cranky because of some disappointment, an offer of an ice cream cone or a cookie solves the problem. Or does it, really? The problem is solved for the parent, maybe, but not for the child. If the child does not find another way to handle the emotion, then food becomes the way; often the only way. And the fat cells enlarge and multiply.

How do you know if you have developed a pattern of using food to solve emotional problems? By monitoring yourself. By reflecting upon, arranging and developing your thoughts during the day, particularly those which are food related. A quiet room and a comfortable chair are conducive to reflection.

The notebook you prepared in the last chapter will provide a convenient way of recording your feelings at the moment of making an eating decision, to see if a thought pattern is revealed.

Ground Rule Number Six is to monitor your thoughts, feelings, attitudes, and emotions before going on, and while you are on the One-Day-At-A-Time program. If this monitoring produces no such pattern, you are emotionally in the clear. If a pattern is evident, then a simple Mental Plan will become part of your One-Day-At-A-Time Plan. That is one way *your* "book" will be especially helpful.

More about the Mental Approach later. Let me just say now that it involves learning to know and understand yourself and taking better care of your needs and wants. For instance, if you are lonely, the refrigerator is poor company. You owe yourself more than that. Extra trips to the refrigerator lead to obesity, and obesity only leads to greater loneliness.

You are going to pamper yourself on the Mental Plan. You are going to give yourself what you really need.

The Unexpected Benefits That Come with Weight Loss, and Sooner Than You Think

Pilots follow ground rules—and air rules. I want to tell you a story of a pilot who had to stop flying when he grew too big for the cockpit and an unexpected benefit he received.

Ground Rules for the One-Day-At-A-Time Plan

When Roger K. was a fighter pilot in the Air Force, he treated himself to four or five huge meals a day. In fact he left the service weighing 230 pounds—nearly 50 percent more than when he enlisted. As a fighter pilot, he was always the first to spot an enemy aircraft. He built a reputation of being the top man in his squadron.

As it became increasingly difficult to squeeze into the cockpit, he found other changes were taking place. His eyesight was not as good, and he was becoming overly cautious; not a good characteristic when you are involved in air combat with a desperate enemy. Because of his increasing weight and decreasing vision, the flight surgeon pulled him off flight status and gave him a desk job. And that is the way he left the service.

He did not resume flying until ten years later; meanwhile he was doing jobs he disliked, Finally, he had a chance to teach flying and air acrobatics. He received his civilian ratings, subject to his wearing glasses. He realized this career, too, would be in jeopardy if he did not lose weight. He came to me for help.

The Schiff Plan seemed complicated to him at first. He explained, "I decided to keep my lecture notes with me and read them constantly. I just followed instructions and the rest automatically handled itself."

He lost 15 pounds in one month. Then something strange happened. I'll let Roger tell you:

"One day as I approached Santa Paula Airport, I looked at the instrument panel to check my altitude. I could not read the meter. I had to take off my glasses. Then I could read it clearly.

"This aroused my curiosity. I decided to leave them off and peered over the cowling for a glimpse of the runway. Actually, in my excitement about seeing without my glasses, I had overflown it. There was the California Trout Hatchery at Fillmore which I knew to be ten miles beyond the airport. I made a 180° turn and could easily see the runway. It was a clear black strip. Still with no glasses on, I could read the '22' that marked its beginning. I judged my landing perfectly. My depth perception was right on the button. I set her down right on those numbers and came to a stop with half the runway to spare."

Roger can now both drive and fly without glasses. That 15-pound weight loss has been followed by another 15 and another. He feels confident in himself and, free of extra ballast, knows he will soar to new peaks in the enjoyment of life.

I do not guarantee you better eyesight by following the One-Day-

At-A-Time Plan and its ground rules. But I do promise you unexpected benefits. And when you follow Ground Rule Number Six, monitoring your thoughts and emotions, one of those benefits may well be insight.

That insight will shed pound after pound with no willpower and with minimal effort. You will be surprised at the needle on the scale because you did not knowingly follow the program, yet lost another pound or more. *Insight gained equals pounds lost.*

"Wait," you say, "What has insight to do with calories?"

Plenty.

Once you recognize false hunger and realize that you actually are not hungry at certain times when you think you are, then appetite has been unmasked. It is like midnight at the masquerade ball and off comes the mask. The one you were dancing with, who you thought was Appetite, turns out to be Insecurity. Well, if Insecurity put on the Appetite mask again, you would not be fooled for a moment. Once false hunger is unmasked, you do not automatically move to the refrigerator for that leftover pie. These 300 or more calories will never be seen on your body.

Insecurity is not a pleasant companion. Neither is loneliness, worry, nor any of the other emotional culprits. Later I will show you an easy way to dismiss these unwanted companions and substitute more desirable emotional company in their place. Beware of the company you keep.

Meanwhile, you can start Ground Rule Number Six immediately. Ground Rule Number Seven gives you a "cage" in which to imprison the culprits.

How Writing Makes Things Right, Especially Weight

As I have explained, you may not be the cause of your overeating. It may have been part of your childhood training or conditioning. But you cannot dismiss the results of that training. Look in the mirror. That extra physical dimension you sport is no fun. It costs you health, sex, money, job, security, and peace of mind, among other things.

It will take an extra dimension to melt away those unwanted bulges—not a physical dimension, but a mental dimension. You need

Ground Rules for the One-Day-At-A-Time Plan

to replace the old, unwanted training with new, desirable training. This is done in several steps:

1. *Monitor* your emotions (Ground Rule Six).
2. *Capture* them on paper (Ground Rule Seven).
3. *Substitute* new emotions and attitudes (later chapters).

Just the way a dream slips away—you think you will remember it but it's gone—so do feelings and emotions slip away. You can identify and cope with these emotions and attitudes by becoming aware of (monitoring) your thoughts.

Many people who use their dreams for personal insight know that they must sleep with pen and paper on the night table and write as soon as they awaken or the dream will not be remembered.

This works too with your monitored thoughts. In fact, it works miracles. Write. Write in your "book." Write to me. Write to yourself. But write! Right now! Writing is Ground Rule Number Seven. It goes hand in hand with Number Six.

Thinking about and recording your thoughts as they occur may seem to have little to do with weight. But just as the presence of nutritious, nonfattening, allowable foods on the plan is a retraining of your eating habits, monitoring and recording your daily thoughts is a retraining of your emotions, attitudes, and thinking habits. It helps to develop the correct mental instructions.

What kind of monitoring and recording? Here is an example. Barbara W. weighed 124 pounds on November 26, 1977. She is five feet two. This is what she wrote then:

WHY I AM FAT

"I am not really fat but I'm not skinny either. Skinny means: sans rolls on the tummy and butt. Skinny, meaning sweaters & slacks, baggy dresses. Without clothes on, now I am GROSS.

"I eat because it feels so good. I put something sweet inside my mouth to shut up the evil words I want to say. To tell my husband he is a fat pig. I eat because I feel so rotten inside thinking he is a fat s.o.b.

"It really is my fault our relationship is failing. I should be willing to work full-time and work at home too. He is a man. It's his right to be around while I work at home. Let him watch TV while I cook, clean, etc.

"I like being fat. I like being ugly because I am so ugly inside.

"My face is ugly anyway, so what does it matter if the rest of my body is too? I've got a hard, thirtyish face. No more softness. New wrinkles every day.

"If I'm skinny, men may like me and I may be tempted to cheat on my husband. I wouldn't *dare* take off my clothes now.

"I'm not getting sex at home. Period. I need comforting. I need loving. Someone to say 'you're not so bad.' So I tell myself I'm not so bad and eat nice sweet things instead. Poor baby, have a cookie."

Some six weeks later Barbara weighed 109 pounds and wrote a letter to herself.

"Dear Barb,

"I'm writing this memo to you so you will not forget about your eating habits. You are a short distance 'Planwise' from your goal of 105 pounds.

"I would like to remind you of several things. First, you were unable to wear any jeans and had to buy dresses. It felt lucky as hell to squeeze into those dresses, with all the rolls of fat surrounding your body. And even worse was bath time—you who love to take baths. You didn't enjoy bathing because you had to fold yourself up to get into the bathtub, all the rolls of fat getting in the way.

"Overeating is like buying something on credit. Tomorrow you have to pay. I know there will be times when you will be possessed with the desire to go on a small binge—but that binge will send you to throwing up because you don't want to regain the weight.

"Binges won't make you feel any better. Momentarily perhaps, but not in the long run."

Now Barbara answers herself:

"The weird part of all this is, I don't want to go off my program. It's not that I want to be skin and bone, it's because I'm enjoying the things I am now eating. I especially remember a Plato salad I ate with cauliflower, broccoli, cheese, salami, onions, lettuce, bean sprouts, tomatoes, celery, carrots, oranges, melon. My taste buds went wild over the tastes and textures. And the chicken breast that I ate last night. It was terrific!

"Well, kiddo, I hope you remember all this stuff. If you ever want to punish yourself again, scrub the floors. Better therapy with good end results!"

Thoughts that were monitored.
Feelings captured on paper.
Weight lost on the scale.
Thus a happier, healthier, slender person.
I've seen it happen thousands of times.
I wish the same for you.

V

ALTERNATIVE DAYS FOR EATING WELL ON THE PLAN

Let us say you have finished reading this book; you are writing in your notebook; and you are ready to begin the One-Day-At-A-Time Plan.

What do you eat?

The answer is: anything you would like to eat, except the disallowed foods. The allowed foods and disallowed foods include all the foods mentioned earlier. There are no "maybe" foods.

It would be advantageous now for you to review those two lists in Chapter III. Repetition is extremely important in the learning process.

In this chapter I am going to help you plan your One Day. I'm also going to help you plan additional days should you decide to repeat the One Day. Before I do this, however, I want to take you through an intensive training course on how to recognize the two most dangerous ingredients to your success. They are carbohydrates and fats.

You are going to be able to spot these two enemies a mile away. Then you can readily eliminate these fattening culprits. You are going to be able to plan, shop, cook, eat, and lose weight with a new concern for your enjoyment, your health, and your peace of mind.

Let's begin with carbohydrates.

Sugar Is Public Enemy No. 1

Periodically the Federal Bureau of Investigation posts lists of the most wanted criminals in the hope that people will help to flush them out of their hiding places.

Sugar deserves to be on that list. And you need to flush sugar out of its many hiding places and down the drain into the sewer where it belongs. Good riddance.

Sugar is an insidious killer. It sings a sweet song as it lures you to your fatty fate. That fate can be as critical as acute obesity, a heart attack, a stroke; or as superficial as mild overweight, a slight muscle strain, or a toothache. Critical or superficial, it is important and meaningful to you.

Sugar comes in several forms. The most common are sucrose, refined from sugar cane or beets; lactose, contained in milk products; and fructose, found in most fruits.

We will learn to spot sucrose like a bloodhound and avoid it like the plague. We will address ourselves to the other two with respectful moderation.

Develop awareness of what you eat. Think before you eat. Think while you're eating.

You have some sugar in your sugar bowl right now. If you toss it away, bowl and all, you have solved only a fraction of the problem.

Some 70 percent of the sugar you consume is hidden. If you could toss away this hidden sugar, too, you would be throwing out about a 125-pound bag of the poisonous white stuff a year. That is the present average consumption of sugar by Americans, up 40 percent since the turn of the century.

All of this sugar you consume in a year, in the sugar bowl or hidden, totals about half your daily carbohydrate calories. Aside from the dangers to your health, do you see now why I am so anxious for you to become aware of sugar's hiding places? Here are just a few, with their total sugar equivalents.

Chewing gum. Every time you take a stick of average chewing gum, it is like taking a half teaspoonful of granulated sugar.

Cola drink. Every time you drink a 6-ounce bottle or glass—you are consuming over 4 spoonfuls of granulated sugar.

Other sweet carbonated beverages. Over 3 teaspoonfuls of sugar in each 6-ounce portion.

Strawberry jam. Jam-packed. Each tablespoon of jam is equivalent to a tablespoon of sugar.

Chocolate cake—6 teaspoons of sugar in a 4-ounce piece, and you can add 4 more teaspoons of sugar for the icing, making a total of ten.

Cup cake (iced)—6.

Brownie—3, unfrosted.

Fig newton—5 teaspoons of sugar.

Doughnut—3 plain; 6 glazed.

Ice cream soda—5.

Ice cream cone—3.

Fruit cocktail—5 in a half cup.

Rhubarb, stewed—8 in a half cup.
Figs, dried—2 in each small fig.
Marshmallow—1½ in each.
Lifesavers—⅓ in each.
Fudge—9 in a 2-ounce square.
Peanut brittle—7 in 2 ounces.
Orange juice—2 in ½ cup.
Pineapple juice—2½ in ½ cup, unsweetened.

Do you see the picture? Do you see why certain nutritious foods such as raisins and apples must remain on the disallowed list? Raisins contain the equivalent of 4 teaspoons of granulated sugar for every ¼ cup you munch. An apple—2 teaspoons of sugar.

It hurts me to banish the apple. It is good for you—unless you are overweight or the pointer on the scale pauses indefinitely in its descent.

How can the equivalent of 3 teaspoons of granulated sugar fit into one tablespoon of something else? It does in honey. As you know, 3 teaspoons equal one tablespoon. Honey is pure sugar. So are molasses, corn syrup, and a variety of flavored syrups.

One tablespoon of maple syrup actually contains the equivalent of 5 teaspoons of granulated sugar because it is more concentrated than sugar.

What about sherbet? It has a reputation of being less fattening than ice cream. Yet, some varieties contain more sugar. Ice cream has one teaspoon of sugar per ounce. Some sherbets have more than 2 teaspoons of sugar per ounce.

An average slice of pie can have the equivalent of anywhere from 5 to 10 teaspoons of sugar, and if it is raisin pie, make that 13 teaspoons of sugar. And if it is à la mode—oh boy!

This is what overweight is all about.

Eliminate this sugar, and you are on your way to slender attractiveness, more business and social acceptance, a healthier and longer life. Also a more joyful and happier you.

White Flour Is Public Enemy No. 2

Flour is easier to spot than sugar. You know it is in bread and everything in the bread family. You know that french toast is flour.

Crackers are flour. Muffins are flour. Cakes, cookies, pie crusts are usually pure white flour, meaning pure poison to the overweight person.

But flour can hide, too. It can hide in soups and stews as thickening. It can hide in coatings used for frying and baking. It can hide in foods with different names such as farina, macaroni, pastas, noodles, and so forth.

The cells of your body feel "left out" every time you eat a product made of white flour. White flour has been "cleansed" of all its natural nutrition. Why? So it will last longer. Insects avoid white flour because it has little food value. Thus, it can be stored for long periods of time without loss to the merchant.

But it is a loss to you of nutrients your body needs. Your only gain is weight. Health and longevity are your losses.

Flour and sugar go through the same metabolic process. In effect, flour is converted to sugar. Flour and other pure carbohydrates, such as sugar, do more to you than supply excess fuel which must be stored as fat. They trigger eating behavior cycles that tend to perpetuate themselves.

Many individuals jump to the conclusion that 250 calories is 250 calories. From a fat storage point of view they mistakenly think it does not matter whether it is 250 calories in a candy bar or 250 calories in a turkey breast.

But there is a difference. You might say there are three significant differences:

1. The turkey, being protein, requires more calories to metabolize than candy. The net result is fewer calories stored.

2. Protein speeds up metabolism while carbohydrates slow it down. The net result is again fewer calories stored when you eat the turkey.

3. Sugar, and to a degree flour, triggers a blood sugar cycle. It makes you feel good for a while, but then comes a letdown which you misinterpret as hunger.

This latter effect, known as the hypoglycemic cycle, results from high blood sugar after eating sweets and starches. This triggers the pancreas to release insulin to neutralize the excess blood sugar. The drop in blood sugar leaves you feeling tired, so you eat even though you have no real need of food.

Selecting Foods for Enjoyment, Nutrition, and Weight Loss

"Have a pretzel?"
"No thanks."
"How about a hot roll, madame?"
"No thanks."
"Would you care for an after-dinner mint, sir?"
"No thanks."

Learn to say "no thanks." Say it to sweets and starches when offered by friend, host, or waiter. Say it to sweets and starches when you pass the coffee shop, the bakery, the ice cream parlor, and all the shelves stocked with fattening items in the supermarket.

"We have fresh halibut today, sir."
"Good, I'll have it."
"Join me for a few leftover chicken legs in the refrigerator."
"Great idea. Count me in."
"The leg of lamb is on special today, madame!"
"Super, weigh this one for me."

Learn to say yes to protein. It certainly says yes to your health. And, it is a definite yes in your weight-loss program.

In some parts of the world, they have pushcarts with meat snacks, but they are not wrapped in bread as are hot dogs and hamburgers.

Instead, they are served on skewers and little sticks. Teriyaki steak bits and chicken bits are common in Japan. In Indonesia, Malaysia, and Thailand street vendors sell saté, which is similar, and in the Middle East they sell kabobs or skewered meat.

There are few carbohydrate calories in these delicious snacks and there is much less of an overweight problem in these countries when compared to the United States. Although we live in a land of abundance, our food intake is all too often abundantly atrocious.

A gourmet meal is not as quick and easy to prepare as a simple snack, a fatty hamburger or a calorie-loaded frankfurter. Yet quick and easy preparation can lead to a quick and fatty demise. You'll eventually acquire efficient and correct cooking habits as you plan your One-Day menus. Perhaps it won't be quick but it will be time well spent. You will be cooking with extra meals and snacking in mind—and with you in mind.

Alternative Days for Eating Well on the Plan

You will bake and roast more, so there will be leftovers. A slice of roast veal, a cold chicken wing, a nibble of leg of lamb, etc. These nutritious, allowable snacks will help you lose weight with ease.

By eating in an enjoyable and sensible way, the one day of selective eating will automatically reach into the next day. You will continue to lose weight, even though you are not formally on the Plan that next day.

Changes take place on the One-Day-At-A-Time Plan that may differ for different people.

Here is how it affected Elise D., a college professor, 43, five feet four, and weighing 143 when she first came to my office. I'll let her tell you in her own words.

"Most of my life I was thin. I had to be careful about my food intake, but I managed to keep my weight at about 114 lbs. Then a trio of events seemed to conspire to cut down on my activity. As a college professor, it was necessary for me to spend many hours reading and typing lecture notes. Then I had a hysterectomy and finally I sprained my ankle. My weight began to increase about two pounds a month until I reached 142. At this point I realized I needed medical assistance and I entered Dr. Schiff's weight-control program. I lost the excess weight in about 6 months, but I had a great deal to learn about eating correctly, and as Dr. Schiff says 'thinking and doing correctly.'

"I continued to keep my weight down until another series of events happened. A promotion in our division opened up. I expected to be promoted as I was the top-ranked professor in the department. I didn't receive the promotion. It went to the newest male member, who was friendly with the V.I.P.'s running the school.

"I was devastated. I cried. I talked with a large number of peole. I gave up in despair and gained back 7 pounds. Finally it struck me that I was letting outside events control my feelings and behavior. I reread parts of Dr. Schiff's lecture notes and concentrated on the meditation aspect of the program. I vowed I would feel happy and be content, not nervous and depressed. I lost the 7 pounds, but a new wonderful feeling came over me—it was almost unbelievable. I began to feel powerful and capable of controlling my own thoughts, feelings, and emotions.

"One day I looked in the refrigerator at a bagel. I actually spoke to the bagel saying: 'Bagel, you can't make me eat you. I decide when and what I'm going to eat. I know I haven't got it made yet, because I'm still snacking after dinner. I recognize that I'm not really hungry when I do this. I feel bored and lonely as my husband is working nights now. I'm going to learn to control this type of eating, too.'

"Some of the progress I have made is in the complete elimination of many disallowed foods from my daily intake. I haven't eaten butter for 6 months. I don't eat cookies, cake, or other sweets. I 'junked' all the junk foods. I eat mainly poultry and fish and have come to really enjoy fresh vegetables and allowed fruits. I like my salt substitute and find normally salted foods unpleasant.

"Some of the physical benefits I have acquired on the weight-control program are lowered blood pressure and greater energy level. My clothes changed from 12-14 to 10. I'm almost a size 9 now. For the first time in my life I'm able to refrain from biting my nails.

"I have a renewed confidence that I can cope with whatever life has to offer. I can handle difficult teaching schedules with equanimity. *More and more, I'm taking and doing one day at a time. There is more truth to that old adage than one can imagine. Although I've known about this before, it finally 'hit home.' It's like the dawn of a miracle!* I've started to forget about the past and not fret about the future. I feel more flexible, like I'll just wait and see what happens. I am able to relax and feel at ease. I'm gaining a feeling that I only have to please myself, not the whole world."

So Elise's career improved by continuing on the One-Day-At-A-Time Plan day after day. She felt no pressure about it. Just one day at a time. Nice and easy.

Louise K., 53, stayed on the One-Day-At-A-Time Plan for 60 consecutive days. During that time, she went from 163 to 135 pounds, which her five-foot one-inch frame accommodated much more attractively. Her benefits were different. Here is how she wrote about it in her "book."

"When I first met my husband, nearly 22 years ago, I was a petite 99 pounds. I wasn't skinny by any means, but with my thin bones and small frame, my weight was distributed perfectly. Without any doubt about it, I had a body built for a bikini.

"One year later, wed to a man who enjoyed my Italian cooking (I was born and raised in Rome, Italy), I began to eat when he ate, and soon became accustomed to cooking American recipes. Soon, I preferred American style cooking to Italian.

"My weight remained the same for the following nine years except for the 25 pounds I soon added because of my age. Or, so I thought. My child was born in 1964, and the weight I gained during pregnancy never left me. It was my mistaken belief that the extra weight was due to the new baby. As I grew older in years, my weight problem also grew.

"In 1975, I enjoyed a tremendous Christmas Day feast, weighing 162 pounds. The excess weight made me feel sluggish and without any relief from the aches and pains old age brought me.

"Despite the pleading by my husband for me to go on a diet and lose the rolls of fat that circled my body, I continued to eat whenever and whatever I wanted. Imbedded in my mind was the mistaken belief that my aches, stiffness, and ill-temper was but a sign of my menopause which caught me totally by surprise.

"The first time I became acutely aware of my overweight condition was the night my husband informed me he was sleeping in the spare bedroom. The next night was the same, and soon it became obvious he had no intention of returning to my bed. Imbedded in my mind now was the realization that the excess weight had isolated me from my husband.

"When I asked him why, he bluntly told me, 'First of all you snore like an elephant, and you thrash and kick the covers as though you are having a nightmare.'

"Quite by accident I met a woman who had been going to a weight control doctor who had helped her to shed 43 pounds of excess blubber. When I learned she was almost the same age and had no muscle cramps or ill-temper which accompanies a 'fat' body and a troubled mind, I decided to visit the doctor myself. Soon after my first appointment, during which time he explained the truth about myself and the underlying reason for my obesity, I began to see myself as others saw me. I began to really understand why I allowed myself become obese, and what to do about it.

"After following Dr. Schiff's weight control plan less than two months, I shed 28 pounds, and regained the vigor I had lost. My ill-temper vanished as the pounds slipped away. Three weeks later my husband discovered that my snoring and thrashing at night had ceased, and he returned to his rightful place by my side.

"With the loss of my excess pounds came a completely new outlook on life. I learned that a woman's vigor and sense of humor doesn't vanish with age, and a woman in her fifties can still be as appealing to her husband as the girl next door."

Do you believe Elise or Louise could have remained on the One-Day Plan day after day, one day at a time, if each day was no different than before?

Do you believe they could be gaining happiness on the program if there was starvation instead of eating pleasure?

Do you believe that either could have withstood the pangs of true hunger if they were denied the full spectrum of nourishment as they confined themselves to the carrot sticks and lettuce leaves of other diets?

Of course they could not. Neither could you. No longer will you have to subject yourself to boredom, starvation, malnutrition, and mental anguish. No longer will you have to subject yourself to the frustration of boring, meaningless and repetitious diets.

Here now are some of the typical eating days you can enjoy on the One Day Program—interesting, filling, nutritious, and gratifying.

Ten Typical One-Day Menus

I want you to understand that I never "prescribe" menus for my patients. It's what you cook between your ears that really counts—food for thought. The scales will move when YOU *learn* to move mentally. The pathway to the body is through the mind.

The following menus are not required regimens. They are merely examples of the variety of daily fare you can enjoy on the One-Day Plan. You may select a One-Day menu for your one day of correct food intake. You may select another One-Day menu for whenever you repeat the one day of improved and enjoyable eating (and my bet is that you will want to stay on it). Or you may scan them for the principles involved, then plan your own menus to suit your own tastes and desires.

Please note that one day's menu is designed to provide snacks or additional meals for that day or the next. This makes a slice of steak just as convenient as the slice of pie used to be. This also makes the one-day intake of food more permissive, convenient, and satisfying. It also allows the pointer on the scale to continue its downward swing.

There are additional hints for making menus more interesting, filling, nutritious, and gratifying later in this chapter.

Assuming you are now eating three meals a day, the "Rule of Two" is applied and five daily meals (mini-meals) are outlined. Remember, portions are to be one-half or less than the usual size. If you are hungry, eat more. But question first if it is actually true hunger as opposed to appetite or false hunger created by negative emotional stimuli.

Monday	Meal # 1	Half grapefruit One egg, any style 1 slice whole wheat toast Coffee (decaffeinated, skimmed or non-fat milk optional)
	Meal # 2	Cottage cheese (low fat) with chives Tea (weak—there are many flavored teas, low in caffeine content)
	Meal # 3	Tuna fish salad Dill pickles, radishes Low-calorie soft drink
	Meal # 4	Two deviled egg halves Buttermilk
	Meal # 5	Tomato juice Hamburger steak Mushrooms Broccoli Half grapefruit Coffee (decaffeinated)
Tuesday	Meal # 1	Broiled veal kidneys Coffee (decaffeinated)
	Meal # 2	Melted American cheese on 1 slice whole wheat toast
	Meal # 3	Hamburger steak Mixed green salad with low-calorie dressing Tea (weak)

	Meal # 4	Salmon salad Low-calorie soft drink
	Meal # 5	Broiled chicken String beans Cole slaw Melon Coffee (decaffeinated)
Wednesday	Meal # 1	Tomato juice 2 scrambled eggs Coffee (decaffeinated)
	Meal # 2	1 slice whole wheat toast Buttermilk
	Meal # 3	Broiled pork chop, lean Cole slaw Tea (weak)
	Meal # 4	Cold chicken Low-calorie soft drink
	Meal # 5	Broiled halibut Spinach Carrots Strawberries Coffee (decaffeinated)
Thursday	Meal # 1	Half grapefruit Cold halibut Coffee (decaffeinated)
	Meal # 2	Hamburger patty (specially prepared—sans fat) Tea (weak)
	Meal # 3	Shrimp salad Half grapefruit Low-calorie soft drink

	Meal # 4	Camembert cheese 1 slice whole wheat toast Skim milk
	Meal # 5	Roast leg of lamb, lean Cauliflower Mixed green salad Low-calorie dressing Half grapefruit Coffee (decaffeinated)
Friday	Meal # 1	V-8 Juice Reheated lamb slices Coffee (decaffeinated)
	Meal # 2	Cottage cheese (low fat) Coffee (decaffeinated)
	Meal # 3	Cold shrimp Mixed green salad Low-calorie dressing Tea (weak)
	Meal # 4	Broiled mushrooms on 1 slice whole wheat toast Buttermilk
	Meal # 5	Baked turkey loaf Asparagus Dill Pickles, radishes Melon Coffee (decaffeinated)
Saturday	Meal # 1	Grapefruit juice (fresh) 2 eggs any style Coffee (decaffeinated)
	Meal # 2	Turkey loaf Coffee (decaffeinated)

	Meal # 3	Asparagus on 1 slice whole wheat toast Swiss cheese Low-calorie soft drink
	Meal # 4	Shrimp cocktail Postum
	Meal # 5	Broiled flounder Boiled white onions Watercress 1 plum
Sunday	Meal # 1	Tomato juice Turkey loaf Coffee (decaffeinated)
	Meal # 2	Hard-boiled egg 1 slice rye toast Skim milk
	Meal # 3	Cold flounder Reheated onions Tea (weak)
	Meal # 4	Cottage cheese (low fat) Low-calorie soft drink
	Meal # 5	Sirloin steak, lean Braised celery Mushrooms Blueberries Coffee (decaffeinated)
Monday	Meal # 1	Half grapefruit Cold steak Coffee (decaffeinated)
	Meal # 2	Hard-boiled egg Buttermilk

Alternative Days for Eating Well on the Plan

	Meal # 3	Turkey loaf Mixed green salad Half grapefruit Tea (weak)
	Meal # 4	Green pepper wedges with pot cheese Low-calorie soft drink
	Meal # 5	King crabs Endives String beans Rhubarb Coffee (decaffeinated)
Tuesday	Meal # 1	Chicken livers on 1 slice rye toast Coffee (decaffeinated)
	Meal # 2	Rhubarb Low-calorie soft drink
	Meal # 3	2 fried eggs (no butter or oil) American cheese Coffee (decaffeinated)
	Meal # 4	Mixed salad Tea (weak)
	Meal # 5	Roast squab Cauliflower Honey Dew melon Coffee (decaffeinated)
Wednesday	Meal # 1	Blueberries 1 egg any style 1 slice rye bread toasted Coffee (decaffeinated)

Meal # 2   Pot cheese
           Skim milk

Meal # 3   Cold squab
           Cauliflower
           Tea (weak)

Meal # 4   Deviled egg
           Postum

Meal # 5   Roast veal
           Cabbage
           Gelatin dessert
           Coffee (decaffeinated)

How and What to Switch to Increase the Fun

As you examine these ten days, you see the only real cause for repetition is the economics of food buying and preparation.

If you roast a leg of lamb, you will very likely have lamb left over. This does not mean another evening of roast lamb, but it does add a variety to your other four meals the next day. You can have a few thin slices of lamb for breakfast, heated or cold; also for lunch or either of the two in-between mini-meals. Switch the leftovers you have and switch the meals in which you have them.

Switching food is important. Variety makes for more "kiks"—more enjoyment as well as a full spectrum of nourishing vitamins and minerals.

You switch meat with fish, fish with poultry, poultry with seafood, seafood with cheese, and cheese with fish.

You switch breakfast juice and fruit, eggs and meat. You switch second breakfasts from leftovers to cottage cheese to deviled eggs to broiled mushrooms to chicken livers, and so on.

You never have the same two lunches during any week. Switch from tuna salad to cold chicken to shrimp salad to hamburger patties. Enjoy cold Alaskan king crab or a can of lobster meat, Swiss fondue or melted American cheese.

When one whole-grain loaf is used up on your one slice a day, switch to a different type of whole-grain bread. We went from whole wheat to rye in these menus but, you can go to fiber breads or multigrain varieties.

Switch melons. Switch berries. Switch flavors. Switch drinks.

On the subject of drinks, I assumed that coffee, tea, and low-calorie soft drinks would probably be your choice. However, there are coffee substitutes, such as Postum, and many interesting herb teas.

Vary your vegetables. Try some you are not accustomed to eating.

Vary your salads. There are so many different lettuces and so many different additional ingredients that make healthful salads. Adding watercress to salad or some raw onion or spice decreases the need for dressing, as it gives the salad a tang. So do sliced radishes and green peppers. Use sprouts in your salad. Use raw mushrooms. Use unlimited vegetables, cheese, egg, turkey or chicken, and so on.

Be innovative and adventurous.

Save your one fruit per day for dessert when desired. Fresh is preferred. If canned, eat only those packed in water or natural juice. Use dietetic gelatin desserts. There are recipes using eggs and powdered milk that make tasty desserts, but avoid regular sweeteners. The French frequently eat cheese for dessert. The electric blender can mix cottage cheese and fruit into interesting and delicious creamlike desserts.

But concentrate on meat, poultry, and fish. Let nutritious proteins be the focal points of your menu planning.

Leg of lamb is an event.

Roast capon is a festivity.

Broiled mackerel is a celebration.

Roast prime rib of beef is a party.

Make it so.

Make each switch a switch from pleasure to more pleasure.

How to Derive More Satisfaction from Every Bite

You will be eating interesting, filling, nutritious, and gratifying food. I know you are anxious to begin; but hold off for another few chapters, as there are other important aspects to understand in order to fully enjoy and succeed with the One-Day Plan.

It is interesting because it is diversified. It is filling because it is rich in life-supporting protein. It is nutritious because, in addition to the protein, you are nourishing your body with the vitamins, minerals, and nutrients in cheese, eggs, fresh fruits, whole grains, and fresh vegetables. And it is gratifying because it satisfies your true hunger.

Your portions are smaller. Your meals are more frequent. You are drinking at least eight full glasses of liquid a day. Coffee, tea, juice, and low-calorie soda count toward this quota, but don't ignore water. Have a few tall glasses a day. Water helps to break up the acid (ketosis) that is a product of protein metabolism.

Each day you opt for the one day of improved and satisfying intake (eating allowed food, not overeating) you will lose weight. Continue with it day after day, one day at a time, and you will lose pound after pound. It is that simple, yet different. It is that effective, yet permissive.

Do I have to tell you what excitement you experience as you see a slender, elegant new you in the mirror when you arise each morning?

It would not be that exciting, and you would not look that elegant and slender if you were bored instead of interested, starved instead of satisfied, nutritionally deficient instead of fully nourished, or anguished instead of gratified.

This exhilaration at the sight of yourself, without having to pay for it in pain and deprivation, is worth a few more easy steps. These steps work even further toward your interest, satisfaction, nutrition, and gratification.

Just as the one day of correct and enjoyable food intake is a switch from sugar, starch, and fat to protein and other nutrients, so it is a switch from one kind of eating behavior to another kind of eating behavior.

Make these slenderizing behavioral switches and you increase, not decrease, your eating enjoyment. Conscious, aware eating is several times as enjoyable as automatic, unaware eating; therefore less fattening.

Watch a lunch counter some day at noon. See how some people sit down, order a hamburger, a piece of pie topped with ice cream, and a cup of coffee with cream, wolf it down, light a cigarette, pay their check, and leave. Many cannot remember how that hamburger tasted. They are deficient in "kiks." They are going to look for "kiks" later, hungry or not. And they are going to gain weight despite their many impassioned excuses, "I tried to resist the food," "I love food and sweets," and so on.

You can obtain more "kiks" out of eating as you lose weight, *if* you make some additional switches.

How to Switch Mannerisms and Habits in Ways That Pay Off in Pounds Off

One of the most common mistakes of the overweight person is to skip meals. Such a person is like the runner who skips several workouts until the day of the race. Breakfast skipped is like saying, "Ready!" Lunch skipped is like saying, "Get set!" And at five o'clock comes the thunderous roar of "Go!" What follows is a nonstop marathon of eating from cocktail snacks through a heavy dinner, through after-dinner munching, through a midnight snack or two. Or three?

Poor body. All that food at one times requires the body to store it, then develop additional blood capillaries to supply the expanded fuel depots. This places a strain on the system and vital organs, frequently leading to health problems such as elevated blood pressure and cardiac abnormalities.

All this eating is done at a time when work is finished and less fuel is needed, not more. So the body must store most of that food as fat.

Switch.

The presence of food, the sight of food, the smell of food, coupled with disturbed emotions and negative attitudes can trigger a feeling of hunger which is not true hunger. It is appetite.

Learn to cope with, curb, and control your appetite (false hunger), your feelings and emotions.

Learn to recognize and satisfy true hunger.

Self-learning equals "self-instructing."

Have two mini-breakfasts, two mini-lunches, and taper off in the evening.

Have more, not less. But have it earlier in the day when the body needs fuel. Let the fat storage cells in your body take a vacation.

That is why the "Rule of Two" works. This is why two *more* meals daily takes weight *off*, and having fewer meals daily can increase your weight.

So here is an important switch to make: Switch from more food at the end of the day to more food at the beginning of the day.

Another advantage of the "Rule of Two" is the "kiks" build-up that five mini-meals provide as opposed to three regular meals. An overweight person, especially one on a standard diet, is tempted much more than the slender person by the sight and smell of food. The sight of those doughnuts in the shop window can "get to you" a lot easier when there are long intervals between meals. Permitted snacks between meals will help you avoid these "fattening sights."

Recognize these cues for what they are—the emotional and impulsive need to eat when you have no real hunger at all.

Muse about these cues. Choose instead to lose.

The switch:

Switch from emotional and impulsive tasting of what you see or smell to what you have consciously planned to eat. Make a daily menu.

Another characteristic of the overweight person is to eat rapidly. When you eat rapidly, you lose "kiks" and gain weight. Which would you rather have? If you vote "no" for the weight and "yes" for the "kiks," then you must switch from fast to slow eating. You must go into slow motion. Slow down the action the moment you sit down at the table. Relax. Easy does it. Uneasy *doesn't* do it.

Pick up and unfold your napkin slowly. Pick up your knife and fork slowly. Take smaller mouthfuls. Chew slowly. Reflect upon your food as you chew. Don't take another forkful until you have swallowed whatever is in your mouth. Enjoy.

The switch:

Switch from your present eating pace to a much slower pace. Savor every mouthful. Treat it like a friend you hate to see leave.

Now here are additional switches that will pay off in pounds off. Some may not apply to you, but if the shoe fits, wear it. It will prove to be a smaller size shoe:

Switch from talking while you eat to talking only between mouthfuls.

Switch from rapid, nonstop eating to placing your spoon or fork down momentarily.

Switch from drinking beverages rapidly to sipping beverages.

Switch from cleaning your plate to leaving something on your plate.

Alternative Days for Eating Well on the Plan

Switch from large to small dinner plates.

Switch from eating anywhere in the house—such as standing in the kitchen, or sitting watching television, or talking on the phone—to eating only while at the one table.

These are small switches to make, but you are switching to a smaller you—day by day.

Take a page of your "book" now and write about the many switches or alternatives that will give you more time to enjoy your regular plus two extra mini-meals.

Write a list of switches or food alternatives similar to those I have mentioned. Spot a few I didn't mention that apply especially to you. Include them on your list. Also, on another page, write a planned One-Day menu of allowed foods with the two extra mini-meals. Make it a delicious day. Make it an enjoyable day. Make it the One Day.

The next chapter is a cooking chapter. How to cook for more "kiks," more nutrition, more belly-full satisfaction, and a more slender you.

VI

DOCTOR SCHIFF'S PRESCRIBED EATING DAY

"Doctor Schiff, I have decided to go on the One-Day-At-A-Time Plan for one day. Please give me your prescribed menu for that day."

In this chapter, I am going to "prescribe" the one day of correct and improved eating for you. However, it will not be a menu. It will be a day, repeated as often as you wish. The One Day, which includes an improved and satisfying intake of food, is an important part of the One-Day-At-A-Time Program.

It will not be a typed sheet showing you exactly what to eat for breakfast, lunch, and dinner. That would make it a formal diet, which it definitely is not. It will be a chapter explaining and suggesting what to eat, drink, think, and do—one day at a time.

I am going to assume that before reading this chapter you have covered the preceding information conscientiously enough to have your notebook started and to know basically what allowed and disallowed foods are on the One-Day plan.

I am going to assume, too, that before beginning this One Day—the first day of the rest of your more slender and enjoyable life—you will have completed reading this book.

A Before-Breakfast Procedure That Helps Your Day Go Well

You awaken. It is the day after completing this book and you are "rarin' to go." Your One Day has arrived.

Don't jump out of bed yet.

Stretch. Relax. Stretch again.

Stretch the way you have seen a cat stretch. Limber up the muscles and tendons. Start the circulation flowing.

Stretch your back, your legs, your arms.

Now place your feet on the floor and remain seated at the side of your bed for a moment. You still feel relaxed and a bit sleepy.

Think about the kind of a day this is going to be. Review in your mind the following happenings in their chronological order.

See (visualize, imagine) yourself eating breakfast. Go over each item of food: the half grapefruit, the soft-boiled egg with one piece of whole wheat toast, the coffee (black or non-fat milk added, no sugar).

See yourself satisfied with this breakfast and not finding it necessary to eat until the next meal.

See yourself on time in anything you have to do during the day, with no stress or tension due to the clock.

See your relations with other people at work, on the phone, at home, and in all your activities during the day, as progressing harmoniously. See yourself smiling. See others reacting positively to you. See yourself reacting positively to you.

See all of your meals taking place at their proper time, just as you have planned, with no sweets, starches, or fat, no disallowed foods. See yourself receiving a parade of "kiks" from these meals, then being thoroughly satisfied and content with no need to eat between meals.

See the remainder of the day going well. See yourself successful, radiant, already beginning to look more slender, already beginning to feel more energetic and youthful!

See and experience your miracle in action.

You are now ready to live the day the way you have reviewed it with your "mind's eye."

How to Start Diminishing Your Measurements

When you have removed your pajamas or nightgown, stand in front of a full length mirror "au naturel."

Take a long look at yourself. Let the look linger in areas you want to change. First look at those areas where fat is being stored. How would you look with five inches off the hips? Would your thighs look more attractive with about two inches off? Abdomen, buttocks, chin? Cover it all. Decide how many inches you will take off each storage "depot." Visualize a scale and see the needle go down as the inches come off. Visualize yourself and see the new, slender, alluring you.

Now cover other physical improvements you would like to make.

Would you like to stand straighter?
Would you like to have a clearer complexion?
Would you like to have a different hair style?
Would you like to have a more youthful appearance?

See the improvements in your imagination. Actually picture them in your mind—flash them onto your "mental screen."

This visualizing of yourself as you want to be is an important step toward reaching your desired goal. Visualization is also an important part of the learning process. Visualization (imagination) plus relaxation, reinforced by repetition *is* the learning process.

Doctors are realizing more and more the important and meaningful part the mind plays in shaping the body. As you think (or don't think), so you are.

You will be monitoring your thoughts today, just as you will be monitoring your food. It will not be "heavy." It will be "light." And you will become lighter with each passing day.

Heavy thoughts promote a heavy body. Light thoughts promote a light body.

Monitor carefully day by day and promote a slender, happier you.

You need to enjoy your thoughts, just as you enjoy your food on this One Day. Both can be "delicious," filled with "kiks."

I prescribe positive thoughts, success thoughts, happy thoughts, joyful thoughts. These are also slenderizing thoughts. Derive "kiks" out of your thinking and achieving, just as you do today out of your eating—and playing—and being.

When you leave the mirror and begin to dress, you realize more than ever, this is really a great day. You know you are in for a turning point in your life. This is like the dawn of a miracle. This is *your* miracle—YOU.

Enjoyment of positive thoughts and actions, and enjoyment of food that is positively nutritional, combine to melt the pounds and inches away—forever.

A Unique Way to Approach Your Meals This Day

You complete your washing and dressing and are ready for breakfast. This is a different day, but you hands do not yet "know" it. They may reach for the cereal bowl.

Understand and learn how to control your hands. They have learned many skills from you—maybe how to sew, drive, write, type. You do not have to guide your hands with these skills any more. They "know" just what to do. In fact, you can carry on a conversation while you sew, drive, write, type.

You have "taught" your hands to go through kitchen procedures too. Let them, and your hands will take you through these same procedures—making the orange juice, pouring the crispy flakes and piling on the sugar.

"Hands," you must say, "this is a different day." Then you must guide your hands to do what you have now planned for your breakfast and for your other meals on this different day.

Cut the grapefruit, boil the water, insert the egg, make the slice of toast, prepare the decaffeinated coffee.

Remember when you last "taught" your hands? You observed every detail of what was to be done, then did it.

Be extra observant now. Notice the grapefruit when you slice it. Is it thick or thin skinned? Juicy or dry? Seeds or almost seedless? Pink or white? Notice the shape of the egg and whether it is medium or large, brown or white. Keep this observation going as you prepare your plate and setting. Maybe, since today is a different day from yesterday, you deserve a different setting; some special plate may be in order, a cup instead of a mug, or a decorative place mat, maybe a linen instead of a paper napkin, perhaps a few candles glowing softly.

Remember now how I told you to derive more satisfaction and enjoyment out of every bite? "Think before and while eating"—remember?

As you begin your breakfast, fix this enjoyment resolve in your mind. Forget the clock. An extra minute or two is really all it takes to convert an automatic breakfast which, ten minutes later, you do not even remember eating, into a breakfast "event."

Start with the first segment of grapefruit. Feel the segment explode its goodness inside your mouth. Feel the tingling aliveness of it. After you swallow, become aware of the change that has taken place in your mouth—the freshness, the awakening of the taste buds, the energizing of your body. Repeat this awareness for each segment. Take no mouthful for granted. Clean the skin, squeeze the last drop of juice from it, maybe even thank it for the pleasure and benefits that you derive.

You can do this with any food. I will not spend more time on this approach to food satisfaction and enjoyment now, but you need to spend a few minutes on this with every bite you take during your four, five, or six mini-meals.

You need to eat with slow motion so as to store up "kiks." Chew slowly, savor every bite, perhaps count your bites.

Although I devote only a few paragraphs to this, Robert Farrar Capin devotes a whole book to it. In "The Supper Of The Lamb," he describes not only how to prepare such a supper but how to prepare to prepare it. He makes a celebration out of a simple supper.

You have a number of celebrations awaiting you today. Celebrate each meal. Celebrate each thought. Celebrate each "kik."

Soon you will be able to celebrate a new, alluring you.

How Recipes Add Joy and Subtract Pounds

If each meal is a celebration, does this mean you have a cake and light the candles?

No, indeed. In fact, no cake is what you are celebrating. Cake brings fleeting moments of sickly sweet mouth pleasure followed by sickly sour years. It also brings sickly excess weight. This in turn brings sickness, dis-ease.

No, we will not celebrate with sweets and limit our pleasure to mouth. We will celebrate with our whole body, mind, and being.

We will celebrate the preparation, serving, ingestion, and digestion of food. We will celebrate the reversal of the weight-adding process. We will celebrate the dawn of a new and better life. We will celebrate a miracle—you.

Let's start with the kitchen. Food needs to be properly stored, prepared, and cooked. Utensils and dishes need to be properly arranged. A table needs to be properly appointed. The mood and surroundings need to be agreeable. These are some of the prerequisites for the true enjoyment of food.

Chaos does not promote festivity. It obstructs progress. Place your house in order, beginning with the kitchen. Be proud to be in your kitchen. Be proud.

Men and women alike are having more fun in the kitchen. There are new utensils and appliances that help us prepare food in interesting ways. There are many mouth-watering recipes that are program oriented.

George M., 67, has taken over the cooking duties for his healthy family of seven. Retired from business, his wife has converted a photography hobby into a successful professional career; so he dons an apron every afternoon and comes up with new dinner casseroles and surprises daily. George did not know how to boil water five years ago. But now he is a source of some of the slimming recipes I share with my patients to provide new ways to make ordinary foods something extraordinary.

George's joy comes from using healthful ingredients—such as natural protein and fresh greens—and cooking them in ways that are unusual, yet retain their vitamins, minerals, and goodness. His joy radiates around the table at every meal. In turn, the table radiates joy.

Innovations in the kitchen transforms boredom into pleasure. Whenever you are creative you dispel boredom. And down the drain together with boredom flow all the negative and unwanted things you do and think about that made you overeat and overreact. In fact, boredom and stress are two significant factors that turn normal people into "excessive" people—excessive with food, liquor, tobacco, and stimulants. Excessive with their emotional being, too.

As your food becomes colorful and cheerful, so do your thoughts. And so do you.

The key is "kiks."

Recipes That Add "Kiks" to Cooking and Dining As You Lose

Here are a number of recipes to help make your One Day a day full of "kiks." You can improve on them, I'm sure. This is just to start you thinking of ways to make each dish an even greater delight. The more you enjoy eating, the more you will lose, because you will want to repeat the One Day again and again.

Soon it becomes a habit to eat in a slenderizing instead of fattening way.

Here are one or more ideas for slenderizing snacks, appetizers, soups, entrées, salads, desserts, and beverages. When you plan your menus for this One Day, include one or more of these, changed as you wish.

You don't have to stop with these alone. There are numerous recipes and ideas in cook books, magazines, and local newspapers that are program oriented. If you wish, your daily menus can be a gourmet's delight.

Apologies to my patients if I have divulged any family secrets and, at the same time, accept my thanks for your sharing with others.

t = *teaspoon*
T = *tablespoon*
C = *cup*
subst. = *substitute*

APPETIZERS

Carrot Curls: Cut a thin strip of carrot with a sharp-edged knife. Wrap each slice around your forefinger and stick a toothpick through the unwrapped curl. Chill on ice to curl, then remove toothpick.

Celery Frills: Cut cleaned stalks of celery into three-inch strips. Cut lengthwise into very thin strips from both ends, leaving about one-half inch of uncut portion in the middle. Chill on ice until they curl.

Radish Roses: Trim stem and cut off root end. With tip of sharp knife cut 3 or 4 tiny pieces from outside red skin, then cut outside the red skin down from the root end toward stem in four different sections to form petals. Chill on ice to open.

Radish Fans: Trim off root end and leave one-inch stem. As for radish roses, starting at one side, cut thin slices toward the stem end, being careful not to cut all the way through. Chill on crushed ice to open.

Cucumber Scallops: Score outside of cucumber by running tines of a fork down cucumber. Slice very thin and place on ice to crisp.

Boiled Shrimp

½ lb. shrimp
1 bay leaf
2 sprigs dill
1 qt. water

Wash shrimp well. Bring water to boil with the herbs. Drop in shrimp and cook till pink. Remove shells and veins. Leave tails on for easy handling. (About ten minutes cooking time.) Makes 2 servings.

Stuffed Mushroom Caps

8 large mushroom caps
1 clove garlic
½ C skim milk
½ onion

Stems from caps
½ t paprika
Salt (or subst.) and pepper to taste

Rub caps clean with damp cloth. Lay in pan and cover with ¼ C skim milk or water. Cook in double boiler or bake until soft. (Bake the stems also.) Save the liquid. Dice onion and mix with mashed garlic. Brown in 2 T skim milk under the broiler. Save liquid. Mix with the stems. Moisten with remainder of milk. Mash. Heap into mushroom caps. Top with paprika. Line shallow pan or baking dish with liquid in which mushrooms were cooked. Bake or broil five minutes. Serve hot.

Baked Brown Eggs

1 dozen eggs, in shell
1 t chicken bouillon powder dissolved in ⅔ C hot water

3 T oil (safflower)
3 small onions, with peel
1 garlic clove, peeled

Put all the ingredients in a baking pan. Bake at 225 degrees 10-12 hours or overnight.

SOUPS

Tomato Soup

2 quarts beef stock
8 medium sized tomatoes, peeled
2 C celery, sliced
¼ C chopped fresh parsley
1 t salt (or subst.)

1¼ t thyme
2 bay leaves, crumbled
1 garlic clove, crushed
½ t mustard seed
Chopped fresh parsley to garnish

Place all ingredients in a large pot and bring to a boil over high heat. Skim the surface and reduce heat. Cover and simmer 45 minutes. Strain liquid into large bowl; discard the bay leaves and purée vegetables in food blender. Stir purée into liquid and cool. Garnish with chopped parsley. Makes 10 servings.

Asparagus Soup

1 beef bouillon cube
1 C hot water
1 (19-ounce) can asparagus
1 large can string beans
½ t onion salt (or subst.)
¼ t pepper

Dissolve the bouillon cube in hot water. Blend all the ingredients (including liquid on asparagus and beans) in blender. May be served either hot or cold.

Cucumber Soup

2 C grated cucumber
¼ C finely chopped onion
1 t sugar subst.
1 t salt (or subst.)
½ t ground black pepper
1 t dried dill
2½ C water
2 cans condensed beef bouillon
2 T lemon juice

Combine the cucumber, onion, sugar subst., seasonings, water, and bouillon in saucepan. Simmer for 10 minutes. Stir in lemon juice and serve. Excellent if served chilled. Yields 8 to 10 servings.

ENTREES

Chicken Supreme

1 broiler-fryer chicken cut into serving pieces
1 t salt (or subst.)
1 t paprika
¼ t pepper
2 T salad oil (safflower)
¼ t turmeric
¼ t ground cardamon
¼ t curry powder
⅛ t dry mustard
1 medium onion, sliced
½ C water

Sprinkle chicken (skin removed) with salt, paprika, and pepper. Heat oil in skillet. Place the chicken in the hot oil. Brown on both sides. Add water, spices, and onion. Cover and cook for 30 minutes longer, or until the chicken is tender. Remove chicken to the serving platter. Spoon sauce over chicken. 6 servings.

Pan Broiled Flounder

4 small flounders	½ t oregano
1 C skim milk	¼ t paprika
1 T vinegar	Salt (or subst.) and pepper to taste

Sprinkle fish with oregano, paprika, salt, and pepper. Cover with milk. Just before serving mix the vinegar into the milk sauce.

Chicken Cacciatore

2½ lbs. chicken, cut into pieces	1 t salt (or subst.)
¼ C oil (safflower)	1 t parsley flakes
1 onion, finely chopped	1 t basil leaves, crumbled
1 garlic clove, minced	¼ t oregano
½ C celery, diced	½ C white wine
2 green peppers, chopped	1 C sliced fresh mushrooms
1 can (1 lb. 12 oz.) tomatoes	Dash of pepper

Brown skinned chicken in hot oil. Remove from pan and set aside. In same oil sauté onion and garlic for 1 minute. Add celery and green peppers and sauté for 5 minutes, stirring occasionally. Add tomatoes (partially mashed). Return the chicken to pan. Season with salt and pepper. Cover and simmer 30 minutes, stirring occasionally. Add remainder of ingredients and simmer 15 minutes longer.

Chopped Meat Patties

1 lb. lean ground beef	¼ C finely chopped onion
1 lb. ground veal	½ C finely chopped green pepper
¼ lb. ground pork (lean)	2 tomatoes
1 C finely chopped mushrooms	Salt (or subst.) and pepper to taste

Combine ground meats, salt, and pepper. Add remaining ingredients, except tomatoes. Shape into 4-inch patties, and fry in coated skillet about 4 minutes each side (or broil). Serve with tomato wedges.

Meat Loaf

1 lb. ground lean beef or half & half beef and veal	2 carrots, grated
	½ t oregano/tarragon
1 onion, grated	½ C onion juice

1 egg (optional)   Salt (or subst.) and pepper to taste
½ t paprika

Add finely grated carrots and onions to meat. Add herbs and seasonings. Break in egg. Mix well in kneading fashion. Bake in Pyrex dish at 375°–400° until done. Baste with a little water and/or onion juice. Serves 4.

Sauerkraut and Meat Patties

½ lb. lean ground beef   ¼ t sage
2 small onions   ½ t thyme
1 egg   ½ t parsley flakes
1 lb. sauerkraut   1 T paprika
1 T skim milk   Salt (or subst.) and pepper to taste
½ carrot, grated

Thinly slice the onions into shallow Pyrex dish. Pour the milk over this and season with salt, pepper, and parsley. Place under the broiler, and keep turning. When brown, remove and add to sauerkraut in juice in Pyrex dish. Bake in 300° oven 15 minutes. Meanwhile mix ground meat with carrots, parsley flakes, sage, thyme, salt, and pepper. Shape into small meat patties (about 8). Roll in paprika. Broil or bake in dish in which onions were broiled. Brown on all sides. Add sauerkraut and onions. Mix well and bake until the mix is brownish.

Marinated Sliced Tomatoes

3 medium ripe tomatoes, peeled   *Exotic Herbs Dressing*
¼ C finely chopped onions

Slice tomatoes into ½-inch slices and place in flat pan. Sprinkle onions and dressing over the tomatoes. Let stand for 1½ to 2 hours, in refrigerator. Separate on plate and cover liberally with juice from pan.

Stuffed Peppers With Mushrooms

6 large green peppers   ¼ t oregano
3 C salted boiling water   2 large onions
Mushrooms, sliced   Salt (or subst.) and pepper to taste
2 C tomato sauce

Soak hollowed peppers in boiling salted water for 5 minutes. Drain. Stuff with mushrooms. Dice onions, add peppers and the tomato sauce. Add oregano, salt, and pepper. Stew or bake, in a covered dish, for about 30 minutes.

Round Pepper Steak

6 oz. round steak cut into slivers	Salt (or subst.) and pepper to taste
1 beef bouillon cube	2 T soy sauce
1 C water	1 thinly sliced green pepper
Garlic powder	

In a nonstick pan, brown steak. Add bouillon cube, water, garlic, salt and pepper, and soy sauce. Cover and simmer for 5 minutes. Add green pepper. Cover, simmer until pepper is tender-crisp.

Spinach Loaf

1 16-oz. carton low-fat cottage cheese	3 eggs
	½ lb. mild Cheddar cheese shredded
1 10-oz. pkg. frozen chopped spinach thawed and drained well	Garlic powder (a little)
	Onion powder (a little)

Mix all together and put into ungreased loaf pan. Bake at 400° for 1 hour or until top is very crispy.

Western Omelet

2 eggs	2 slices cheese
1 T chopped onions	¼ C diced green pepper

Beat egg and onion, let stand five minutes. Heat nonstick pan (or nonstick coating) instead of oil. Add egg mixture and cook. Add cheese and green pepper. Heat until cooked.

Barbecue Sauce

¼ C tomato purée	1 t soy sauce
¼ C water	1 t prepared mustard
¼ t liquid sugar subst.	½ t celery salt
2 T lemon juice	

Mix and simmer for fifteen minutes. Can be used on beef, lamb, or chicken.

Hungarian Goulash

2 lbs. beef stew meat	1 t caraway seeds
1 C thinly sliced onions	⅛ t cayenne
1 can (1 lb. 11 oz.) sauerkraut	½ C chopped green peppers
1 C canned tomatoes	1 C sour cream
1 T paprika	

Cut the beef into one-inch cubes. Brown it on all sides in a Dutch oven. Add onions and sauté until golden brown. Add sauerkraut, tomatoes, paprika, caraway seeds, cayenne along with ½ C water. Cover and cook over low heat about 1 hour. Add green peppers. Cook about 10 minutes longer. Remove 1 cup of liquid. Gradually add the sour cream, stirring so it will not curdle. Pour mixture back into pan.

Chili

1 lb. ground chuck or sirloin	2 T chili powder
¼ C chopped onions	¼ t cumin seed
4 oz. tomato sauce	1 T beef bouillon powder, dissolved
½ t salt (or subst.)	in 2 C boiling water

Brown the meat and onions together and cook until meat loses all red color. Add the chili powder. Stir. Add bouillon and tomato sauce. Cover and simmer 1 hour.

Chili Relleno Casserole

1 7-oz. can whole Ortega Chilies	3 eggs
¼ lb. Jack cheese	¾ C non-fat milk
¼ lb. Cheddar cheese	

In a 9 × 9 square pan, layer ½ of the chili peppers (split open), cover with chunks of Jack cheese, another layer of chilies, then chunks of Cheddar cheese.

Beat eggs with milk. Pour over chilies and cheese. Bake at 400° for 45 minutes or until firm and lightly brown on top.

Ratatouille Pie

1 eggplant, peeled and chopped	1 onion, chopped
2 large zucchini, chopped	4 tomatoes, cut in small pieces

Garlic powder to taste
3 eggs
¼ C parsley
¼ C oregano
¼ t basil
¾ C Parmesan cheese
½ lb. sliced Mozzarella cheese

Put eggplant, onion, zucchini in a frying pan. Cover and simmer on low heat, mix often until vegetables are soft. Add tomatoes and cook a little longer. Season with garlic powder.

Beat eggs, add parsley, ¼ C Parmesan cheese, basil, and oregano. Pour egg mixture over vegetables in frying pan. Cook over medium low heat for several minutes to *set* bottom of eggs. Sprinkle with remainder of Parmesan cheese, cover with sliced Mozzarella cheese. Place in oven under broiler for several minutes until top is browned and puffed. *

Seafood En Coquilles

2 C chopped or shredded boiled shrimp, crab, or lobster meat
1 egg
1 T chopped parsley
½ t lemon juice
1 T ketchup
1 T horseradish
1 T powered skimmed milk
Salt (or subst.) and pepper to taste

Beat egg. Combine with all ingredients but powdered milk. Mix lightly. Fill 4 ovenproof baking shells or ramekins. Sprinkle powdered milk over each. Bake at 375° until brown (10-15 min.).

Zucchini Continental

4 medium zucchini, cut into ¼-inch slices
4 oz. grated Parmesan cheese, reserve 1 T
2 ribs celery, cut into ⅛-inch slices
¾ C tomato purée
½ t salt (or subst.)
⅛ t each pepper, thyme, basil
Dash garlic powder

Preheat oven to 350°F. In an oven-proof 2-quart, nonstick casserole, combine all ingredients; toss lightly. Sprinkle top with reserved cheese. Cover and bake about 25 min. or until zucchini is tender-crisp. Makes 4 servings.

Steamed Vegetables

Steaming is the best and fastest way to bring out the natural goodness and taste plus the fresh flavor of both frozen and fresh vegetables. Water-soluble vitamins and essential nutrients are retained when vegetables are steamed. Also, they are more appetizing and enjoyable.

Place the steamer in a pan, keeping the water level ¼ inch below the bottom of the steamer. Bring water to boil. Place the freshly washed and sliced vegetables on the steamer. Cover the pan with a tight-fitting lid and simmer. Many cookbooks list the steaming time for a variety of vegetables. Vegetables are healthier and more enjoyable when undercooked rather than overcooked. You may mix several vegetables on the steamer without loss of their individual flavor.

For variety—as an example—zucchini may be sprinkled with Parmesan cheese, a little salt substitute, and fresh ground pepper.

Crown Roast of Lamb

1 18-inch crown roast of lamb
¼ t garlic powder
¼ t curry powder
Salt (or subst.) and pepper to taste
Parsley for garnish

Have butcher trim all fat from roast and remove the backbone and French ribs. Place the roast, rib ends up, on rack in roasting pan. Rub combined seasonings over the surface of the roast. Using foil, make a ball and force it into the crown so roast will retain shape while cooking. Cover the ends with foil to prevent charring. Roast, uncovered, for about 20 minutes per pound for medium and 25 minutes per pound for well done in a 300°F. oven. Serve on platter, garnished with parsley.

Beef and Peppers

1½ lbs. lean beef round steak
1 T paprika
2 cloves garlic, crushed
1½ C beef bouillon
1 C sliced green onions with tops
2 medium green peppers, cut in strips
⅓ C soy sauce
3 medium tomatoes, cut in wedges

Pound steak to ¼-inch thickness. Cut across grain in ¼-inch strips. Sprinkle with paprika and let stand about 10 minutes. Place on broiler pan and brown quickly, turning once. Remove to saucepan. Add garlic and bouillon, cover, and simmer about 30 minutes. Stir in onions and peppers; cover and cook 5 minutes. Stir in soy sauce and cook 2 minutes. Add tomatoes and cook until just heated.

SALADS

Seafood Salad

1 C lobster meat, crab, or shrimp
½ C buttermilk
1 T tomato sauce
1 t basil
¼ t garlic powder
½ t soy sauce
½ C chopped celery and green pepper, mixed
Salt (or subst.) and pepper

Shred meat. Add the celery and green pepper. Beat buttermilk with tomato sauce, add the soy, spices, and salt. Pour over seafood and toss lightly.

Cabbage Carrot Salad

3 C shredded cabbage
½ C minced green pepper
3 carrots, grated
1 apple, diced
½ C low-calorie dressing

Combine all ingredients and toss lightly.

Cucumber Salad

1 large cucumber, sliced thinly
1 small onion, sliced thinly
⅔ C wine vinegar
¼ t salt (or subst.)

Combine all ingredients in a bowl. Cover and marinate in the refrigerator for 2 hours.

Chef's Salad Chesapeake

1 can (12 oz.) blue crab meat or other crab meat, fresh, frozen, or pasteurized, or
2 cans (6½ or 7½ oz. each) crab meat
Paprika
1 package (10 oz.) frozen asparagus spears
6 lettuce cups
Dressing
3 hard-cooked eggs, sliced

Thaw frozen crab meat. Drain. Remove any remaining shell or cartilage. Flake the crab meat. Cook asparagus spears according to directions on package. Drain and chill. Place 3 asparagus spears in each lettuce cup. Place

⅓ C crab meat on asparagus. Cover with approximately 2 T dressing. Top with 3 slices hard-cooked egg. Sprinkle with paprika. Serves 6.

Seafood Antipasto

1½ lb. fish filets (canned)	18 celery sticks
2 cans (4 oz. each) button mushrooms	12 radish roses
6 large lettuce leaves	12 tomato wedges
1 cucumber, sliced	6 green pepper rings

Drain fish filets and mushrooms. Place on lettuce leaves. Arrange vegetables around fish filets (with mushrooms in center of plate). Serves 6.

Tuna Salad

1 6½-oz. can dietetic tuna	2 T skim milk
1 5-min. egg	¼ t ground dill seed
1 t mustard	2 stalks celery
1 t wine vinegar	1 small onion
Salt (or subst.)	Pepper

Mash *yolk* with mustard, vinegar, dill, salt and pepper. Grate in onion. Add milk and beat vigorously with *silver fork*. Add tuna and mix. Grate in egg white. Cut in celery. Garnish with tomatoes. Serves 2.

Low-Calorie Dressing

½ C tomato juice	1 T onion, finely chopped
2 T lemon juice or vinegar	Salt (or subst.) and pepper

Chopped parsley, green onion, or dry mustard, etc. may be added if desired. Combine ingredients in a jar with a tightly fitted cover. Shake well before using. Refrigerate.

Buttermilk Style Dressing

1 pkg. seasoning mix, found in local markets, e.g., Hidden Valley, Uncle Dan's, Good Seasons Buttermilk Style, Green Goddess.
1½ C buttermilk
Important—omit 1 C mayonnaise suggested on the package.

Mix ingredients in a jar with a tightly fitted cover, shake well until blended. Refrigerate 12-24 hours before serving to enhance the flavor.

Low-Fat Salad Dressing

1 C low-calorie cottage cheese	¼ t onion powder
2 T lemon juice	1 T minced chives
½ t celery salt	2 T minced parsley
¼ t paprika	

Combine all ingredients in blender and mix thoroughly. Refrigerate.

Dressing For Green Salads

2 T water	½ t liquid sugar (or subst.)
4 T cider vinegar	1 small clove garlic, pressed
½ t salt (or subst.)	½ t grated onion
½ t pepper	

Mix and chill.

DESSERTS

Baked Pears

2 medium pears	Powdered sugar subst.
¼ t powdered allspice	12 cloves
¼ t cinnamon	¼ C buttermilk (optional)

Rub allspice and cinnamon into the pears. Stick six cloves into each. Bake in ½ C water in slow oven, basting often. Sprinkle powdered sugar subst. over pears before serving. Centers may be filled with buttermilk at serving.

Baked Pears

8 pear halves, canned in own syrup	2 cloves
8 T juice	1 t lemon juice
1 t vanilla extract	

Place pear halves in baking dish. Combine pear juice, lemon juice, and vanilla. Pour over the pears. Add cloves and sprinkle fruit lightly with nutmeg. Bake for 30 minutes, spooning juice over the pears occasionally. Serve two pear halves with small amount of juice per serving.

Lime Refresher

1 pkg. diatetic lime gelatin
¾ C hot water
½ C liquid sugar subst.
3 T lemon juice
1 t grated lemon peel
1 C buttermilk
1 stiffly beaten egg white

Dissolve the gelatin in hot water. Add sugar subst. Stir until completely dissolved. Add the juice, peel, and buttermilk. Pour into tray and freeze until firm. Break into chunks and then beat with beater until smooth. Fold in egg white. Freeze until firm.

Frozen Coffee Custard

½ t gelatin
½ C boiling water
1 T lemon juice
5 tablets sugar subst.
½ C strong coffee
¼ C powdered milk
½ t vanilla
1 egg white

Dissolve gelatin in the boiling water. Add ½ T of lemon juice and 2 tablets of sugar subst. Jell to whipped-cream consistency. While gelatin is setting, mix the coffee in which the remaining tablets of sugar subst. have been dissolved with powdered milk and start beating with mixer. While beating add the vanilla, ½ T lemon juice, and a pinch of salt. Beat to consistency of whipped cream. Beat egg white stiff. Beat jellied gelatin into coffee-milk whip and fold in egg white. Put in individual dishes in refrigerator to set.

Coffee Cheese Mold

1 t powdered gelatin
¼ C strong coffee
4 pinches sugar subst.
2 bay leaves
¼ lb. pot or farmers cheese
¼ t vanilla extract

Dissolve gelatin in ¼ C cold water. Add coffee and vanilla extract. Run cheese mixed with sugar subst. through food mill twice. Combine the cheese and gelatin solution. Add bay leaf. Mix thoroughly, dissolve cheese in mix, allowing no cheese particles to remain whole. Remove bay leaf. Pour into molds and chill. Serve on bed of autumn leaves, grape leaves, or chicory.

Gelatin Coffee Dessert

1 envelope unflavored gelatin
½ C cold water
1 T sugar subst.
1 C hot coffee
1 t lemon juice

Soften gelatin in water and stir in the sugar subst. and hot coffee. When completely dissolved stir in lemon juice. Pour into 2 individual molds. Refrigerate. Serves 2.

Fluff Topping

1 C ice-cold skim milk
2 egg whites
30-40 tiny grains sugar subst.
¼ t vanilla extract

Beat milk and egg whites separately to stiffness. Fold together. Add sugar subst. and vanilla. Beat well. Use immediately. This is good over fresh berries, fruits, and drained, water-packed fruits.

Fruit Blend

1 C sliced assorted fruits
1 t brandy extract
1 packet sugar subst.

Combine all ingredients and marinate overnight.

Prune Whip

½ C unsweetened prune pulp*
1⅓ t sugar subst.
1 t vanilla
1 t lemon juice
1 t unflavored gelatin
1 T cold water
2 egg whites

Blend first four ingredients together. Soften gelatin in cold water; then dissolve over hot water. Beat egg whites until frothy; add gelatin and beat very stiffly; fold into prune mixture. Pile lightly into custard cups or sherbet glasses and chill thoroughly.

*You may use 5-oz. jar strained prunes or ¼ pound dried prunes, cooked until soft in ½ C water, then pitted and chopped.

Variation: Apricot Whip—substitute ½ C unsweetened apricot purée for prunes. Serves 4.

Low-Calorie Custard

4 eggs
1 carton (16 oz.) low-fat cottage cheese
1 t vanilla
½ t nutmeg
1 T sugar subst.

Blend all ingredients. Pour into custard cups and sprinkle with more nutmeg. Place in shallow pan in about 1 inch of water. Bake at 325° for 45 minutes. Cool.

Apple Meringues

1 very large apple
1 t powdered skim milk
6 grains sugar subst. tabs
1 egg
¼ t powdered cinnamon

Beat yolk of egg until thick and lemony. Add three grains of sugar subst. and cinnamon. Beat a few seconds. Pare and core apple, cutting into thin slices. Combine with egg yolk. Divide into two portions and fill 2 small individual Pyrex baking dishes. Whip egg white stiff. Add 3 grains of sugar subst., powdered milk, and blend. Top each dish with the mixture. Bake at 350° for 25 minutes.

Spiced Peaches

2 fresh or water-packed peaches
12 whole cloves
¼ t powdered cinnamon
Powdered sugar subst.
½ C lemon or lime juice

Place 3 cloves into each peach half. Cover with juice. Add powdered sugar subst. to taste and powdered cinnamon. Bake in slow oven, continually basting. Add more juice or water if necessary. Serves 2.

Guava Sherbet

⅓ C dry skim milk powder
¾ C water
3 T unsweetened guava juice

Blend all ingredients and freeze in ice-cube tray.

Apple Snow

1 C dietetic canned applesauce	½ t vanilla extract
2 egg whites	¼ t salt (or salt subst.)
½ t sugar subst.	¼ t nutmeg

Add nutmeg, salt, and vanilla to applesauce. Refrigerate until chilled. When ready to serve, beat egg whites until they peak. Add sugar subst. slowly, beating until stiff. Fold in applesauce. Serves 2.

Refrigerator Ice Cream

1 envelope plain gelatin	1½ C whole milk
¼ C cold water	1 C dry milk powder
1 T sugar subst.	1 t vanilla

Soften the gelatin in cold water. After a few minutes dissolve it over heat, stirring. Then stir it into the whole milk. Divide it between two refrigerator trays and place in freezing compartment (normal freezing). When it turns syrupy scrape it into a bowl and beat until creamy. Add the dry milk powder, sugar subst., and vanilla. Beat until the powdered milk dissolves. Return to trays and freeze.

For variations try adding 1 C frozen berries—either strawberries, raspberries, or blueberries.

Pineapple Gelatin Dessert

1 envelope unflavored gelatin	⅔ C hot water
½ C cold water	½ C pineapple juice
1 T sugar subst.	

Soften gelatin in water; stir in sugar subst. and hot water until gelatin is dissolved. Stir in pineapple juice. Pour into two individual molds. Refrigerate until set. Serves 2.

DRINKS

Dr. Schiff's Bloody Mary

3 washed carrots	1 sprig watercress or parsley
⅛ head of cabbage	

Blend all ingredients in juicer.

Dr. Schiff's Thirst-Quencher Slim Fizz

1 freshly squeezed lemon
1 freshly squeezed small lime

Top with club soda

Makes 1 glass.

Dr. Schiff's Hot Toddy

¾ C skim milk
½ t vanilla extract

2 T carob powder

Heat milk. Put carob powder in a mug and add heated milk. Stir in vanilla. Serves 1.

Dr. Schiff's Afternoon Pick-Me-Up

1 (5-oz.) can tomato juice
Worcestershire sauce

⅓ cucumber, cut in chunks
soy sauce

Combine in blender tomato juice, cucumber chunks (leave skin, but if necessary remove seeds). Add a dash of Worcestershire sauce and soy sauce and blend.

Tips for Cooking to Lose Weight

This One Day is a day of enlightenment in the kitchen. It calls a halt to certain fattening practices and encourages you to adopt other slenderizing practices in their place.

It encourages you to fry less and steam more. It asks that if you must fry, use no oil or as little as possible. Instead, coat the pan with Pam, Panstick, Teflon Spray, or a similar product. It asks that you strip fat from meat and skin from poultry and eat around remaining fat.

It asks that you cut down on salt by using a salt substitute. It usually raises an outcry when the family chef is asked to halt salt. But this is helpful to your healthful slenderizing. Salt is mouth pleasure. It is not useful in the body in the quantities we consume.

The body is about 80 percent water. Salt causes the body to absorb even more fluid. When salt is present, pounds go up without excessive food as the cells of the body absorb and retain the water.

Cut out salt and pounds drop away. Your body is less bloated, more flexible. You look and feel better.

"But I can't eat food unless it is salted," you protest. "It's tasteless." Yes, I agree. But there are many salt substitutes that are free of the dangers of salt. I do not recommend Accent or monosodium glutamate. I prefer vegetable salts and sea salts, if you insist on the salt taste. These are available in health food stores. An example is Veg-Salt. There are also a variety of salt substitutes at your local market.

Better yet are the many spices that add zing to soups, stews, roasts, casseroles, salads, and desserts.

Explore the world of spices. Buy some allspice, basil, dill, mustard seed, sage, and thyme as starters. Consult a cookbook or spice book for additional recipes and information on which spice to use, when, and how much to apply. Or experiment for yourself.

Pepper and the other hot spices are fine and nonfattening—a bit irritating to the unaccustomed stomach, but not water-retaining. My objection to the hot spices is that they upstage the others. They overwhelm the taste buds and eclipse the subtle joys available in the spectrum of other spices.

Make changes in the kitchen in this direction. Hide the salt. Begin a spice collection.

Fresh foods in season are tastier and more nutritious than canned foods. Also, the less they are cooked the better. Raw foods have more "kiks" for your cells than cooked foods. Water used in cooking dissolves many nutrients, and they go down the drain with the water. High heat kills other nutrients.

Frozen fruits and vegetables are fine, provided they have been prepared with no additives.

Have a hearty appetite—I mean the real appetite caused by true hunger, not the false appetite caused by false hunger. This false hunger is created by disturbed emotions and negative feelings.

Completing the One Day in a Special Way

A day of fun:

> Fun food
> Fun thoughts
> Fun deeds
> Fun living

You have enjoyed your regular meals plus two.

You have replaced sweets, starches, and fat with meat, poultry, fish and seafood, salads, vegetables, cheese and eggs, fruits, and other allowed foods.

You have eliminated nonallowed foods.

Your thoughts have switched from the heavy, negative, unwanted, fattening thoughts of the left-hand column to the light, positive, desirable, slenderizing thoughts of the right-hand column.

Heavy Thoughts	*Light Thoughts*
Overweight problem	Slender solution
Loneliness	Fellowship
Argument	Understanding
Despair	Hope
Cruelty	Gentleness
Impatience	Persistence
Confusion	Consistency
Harshness	Harmony
Hate	Love
Jealousy	Kindness
Unhappiness	Joy
Deceit	Honesty

It is now time to end your One Day. Do it the way you began.
Sit by the side of your bed.
Relax. Easy does it.
Feel good.
Enjoy.

Doctor Schiff's Prescribed Eating Day

Review the day. Whenever a heavy thought enters this review, switch to a light thought—from negative to positive.

See yourself so immersed in light thoughts that you shine with an aura of light. See the world bathed in sunshine—yours.

See yourself living a pleasant life from now on with wholesome delicious foods and wholesome "delicious" thoughts.

End this pleasant moment with yourself and drift into dreamland.

Pleasant dreams.

. . . And, a slimmer you.

VII

THE AMAZING RULE OF TWO

You are now halfway through the book.

If you were to close this book today and begin tomorrow, would you know exactly what to do to achieve your desired weight?

Well, you would know which foods to eat and which foods not to eat. Perhaps you would be aware of your need to derive more enjoyment out of your food. You would know that your book entitled "ME" plays an important part in the weight-loss program; also, there are other basic elements to the program as spelled out in the preceding chapters.

This is all correct, but now we need to go into details about:

1. The right way to add meals to your day.
2. The right way to cut portions.
3. The right way to switch foods.
4. The right way to switch thoughts, attitudes, emotions and feelings.
5. The right way to instruct your mind how to eliminate unwanted pounds, enjoy *your* life and remain slender forever.

There are right ways and wrong ways to add meals to your day. The rule of two is simple. If you eat two meals a day, add two; that makes a total of four. If you eat three meals, make it five. But what kind of meals? When? It makes a difference—on the scale.

There are right ways and wrong ways to cut portions, switch foods, and switch thoughts. And the technique for instructing your mind to make you slender is an *astounding way* to keep the pounds that roll off permanently off. This technique is, without a doubt, entirely new to you.

That is why you need to delay before beginning your One Day.

Now *that's* unusual, is it not? A doctor who does not say, "I want you to start losing weight immediately and quickly." Instead, I say, "Wait. Have patience. Allow yourself time. Relax.

"And remember to enjoy food more, not less; eat more often, eliminate the mental weight as well as the physical weight; the weight will take care of itself *if* you learn to take care of yourself. You either fail or you make yourself successful, one day at a time."

Your notebook—the book called "ME"—will be your way to successful weight loss and enjoying yourself for the rest of your life.

Even the most widely known approaches to weight loss are rife with failure. A report made to the Second International Congress on Obesity pointed to a 70 to 80 percent failure rate among commercial weight loss groups in the United States, Australia, and the United Kingdom. Margaret Ashwell, Ph.D. reviewed 21 chapters of TOPS (Take Off Pounds Sensibly), Weight Watchers in Australia, Weight Watchers in the United Kingdom, and a number of slimming clubs also in the United Kingdom.

Dr. Ashwell noted that initial weight loss was common but continued weight loss (maintenance) was uncommon. Only 20 to 30 percent attained their recommended weight. There were many backsliders. And, there were many rationalizations and excuses.

The Schiff Plan holds far greater promise for you—successful weight loss and maintenance, day by day.

This promise is not inherent in the specific foods, recipes, or menus. It is inherent in you—your body, yes, but also your mind and your spirit. The complete, Holistic you.

In the last chapter I gave you ways to enjoy the natural goodness of ordinary foods in extraordinary ways—menus that gladden the heart.

In this chapter I give you ways to enjoy food more frequently—more periods each day when the heart is gladdened and the spirit is uplifted.

How to Extract Your Sweet Tooth

Most people who are overweight feel a craving (uncontrolled desire or state of mind, appetite) for sweets, especially sweets combined with flour and/or butter. When they snack, it is usually on cake, pie, or ice cream; candy, danish, or cookies.

When we add a meal we add a really delicious meal, a meal of nourishment, not a meal of sweetness. A hamburger patty. A chicken leg. A fish filet. A steak, etc.

"But I have a sweet tooth," my patients often reply.

Let's extract your sweet tooth now. We won't need a pair of pliers.

We'll just dissolve the myth that there is such a tooth. Do you feel like something sweet right now? Well, set the book aside, but instead of going into the kitchen for a sweet snack, go into the bathroom and brush your teeth. I'll wait. . . . How do you feel now? Certainly not like having a sweet. It is probably the last thing you would want to put in your mouth at the moment.

The craving we have been interpreting as a craving for sweets is really not for sweets. It is a craving for merely a different taste in our mouth. We instruct the mind with each false interpretation, and eventually it becomes a compulsive or impulsive reaction—or a tendency.

You can prove this to yourself by sampling different "tastes" whenever your "sweet tooth" calls out.

Use toothpaste. Use a mouthwash. There are mouth sprays you can carry in a pocket or purse, such as Binaca, which comes in a number of flavors such as "frosty mint."

Eat pickles. Dill pickles or any sour food will put your craving for sweets to rest, fast. Suck a lemon or a lime. Take a drink of water or tomato juice or have half a grapefruit. Sip and savor coffee or plain tea; lemon may be added. Liquid cleanses the mouth and changes its internal environment. The craving for sweets will change, too.

For many, sweets have become such an ingrained habit that changes in taste are not enough to remove the craving (intense, uncontrolled longing; appetite) altogether. If cravings for sweets persist, use sugar substitutes.

A low-calorie gelatin dessert can be stored in the refrigerator for sweet snacking. Change the flavor each time you make it. There is a substitute for chocolate. It is called Carob. It tastes just like chocolate. It comes from the pod of an evergreen tree. It is available in health food stores.

If one of your meals must include a sweet dessert, use a graham cracker crumb crust (roughage) and custard or chiffon fillings. Custard is high in protein. Chiffon is high in air.

There is no such thing as a sweet tooth. There is only a sweet habit. You can cancel the sweet habit by enjoying other tastes instead. Switch. The other foods and tastes then become a new, desirable, slenderizing habit.

How the Two-Meal Person Can Easily Make It Four Meals

Sharon L. gained weight eating two meals a day for years.

Then she lost all the excess weight in a few months eating four meals a day.

Of course, Sharon switched from sweets, starches, and fat to protein as she added the two meals. She also cut portions. Her two meals were lunch and dinner. "I'm too sleepy to eat breakfast," was her rationale.

I convinced Sharon to eat breakfast "just for one day." Her favorite lunch was eggs, so my "pitch" was to have her eat eggs for breakfast instead. I also convinced Sharon to have one lunch in two installments, one at 10 A.M., the other at noon. My "pitch" here was to have her eat her favorite dinner—steak—at lunch and to repeat it at dinner. She agreed.

Sharon added the two meals. She ate breakfast when she arose; she had a cottage cheese preview of lunch at mid-morning. And she had her favorite beef twice a day in different forms. She enjoyed the new routine that day. She enjoyed it immensely, then made a record of her menus so she could follow a similar routine the next day.

Sharon logged a record for eight days, then stopped. The four meal a day routine automatically became her "way." You could say she repeated the Schiff Plan a number of days. But can she or you or I say on which day it stopped being the Schiff Plan and automatically became her "way?"

Here is the record she logged:

WEDNESDAY, 5-21

Breakfast: 2 eggs with cheese, coffee (black)

10:00 a.m.: Cottage cheese (low fat), buttermilk, cucumber slices

12:00 Noon: Steak, lettuce, cucumber, and tomatoes and sauerkraut juice

Dinner: Steak, lettuce, cucumber, and carrots, buttermilk (two small glasses)

THURSDAY, 5-22

Breakfast: Egg, cottage cheese, ground round cooked together
10:00 a.m.: Cheese, milk (non-fat), cucumber, carrots
Lunch: Meat loaf, raw vegetables, buttermilk
2:00 p.m.: Carrot, celery, sauerkraut and tomato juice
Dinner: Chicken, cottage cheese, milk (non-fat), lettuce

FRIDAY 5-23

Breakfast: Two poached eggs
10:00 a.m.: Carrot, celery, cucumber
12:00 Noon: Steak, celery, carrots, cucumber
Dinner: Beef brisket, lettuce, milk (non-fat), and cottage cheese

SATURDAY, 5-24 (Arose late and combined first two meals)

Breakfast: Egg with ground round, cottage cheese, cheese
Lunch: Hamburger patty, tea, carrot, celery
Dinner: Cucumber, cottage cheese, ground round cooked with onions, peppers, and tomato sauce, milk (non-fat)

SUNDAY, 5-25 (Another late morning)

Breakfast: 1 small bowl Special K, with skim milk, coffee
Lunch: Steak, coffee (non-fat milk added)
Dinner: Roast beef, carrots, lettuce, and celery, milk (skim)

MONDAY, 5-26

Breakfast: Eggs with cottage cheese, ground round, coffee (with non-fat milk)
10:00 a.m.: Carrots, celery, cheese
Lunch: Steak, carrots, lettuce
Dinner: Steak, onions, cottage cheese with D-Zerta

TUESDAY, 5-27

Breakfast: Two boiled eggs
10:00 a.m.: Carrots, celery, cheese
Lunch: Hamburger patty, celery, carrots

> *Dinner:* Ground round cooked with onions, tomato sauce, and green peppers. D-Zerta

WEDNESDAY, 5-28

> *Breakfast:* Small bowl Special K, skim milk, one boiled egg
> *10:00 a.m.:* Cheese, celery, carrots
> *Lunch:* Cottage cheese, D-Zerta, celery, lettuce, carrots, and one boiled egg
> *Dinner:* Meat loaf, green salad, D-Zerta with cottage cheese

This food arrangement represents Sharon's preferences. They are not necessarily yours, but they gave her an abundance of "kiks."

The "kik" is more important than the calorie.

When you cut calories and cut "kiks" too, you are in the "diet rut." Soon you'll demand your "kiks." Then the calorie cutting reverses itself, and the weight loss also reverses itself.

When you cut calories and keep or increase "kiks," you never miss the calories you cut because you enjoy plenty of "kiks." Net result: you continue to do what you were doing—losing weight with ease, pleasure, and permanence.

It may have been a regimen that one day. But as you continue with it *by choice*, it is no longer a regimen. It becomes an automatic, enjoyable, and healthful way to eat.

Remember to follow one important principle when applying the amazing "Rule of Two": add meals earlier in the day.

That is why I encouraged Sharon to eat breakfast and a pre-lunch, rather than an afternoon or midnight snack.

Food eaten earlier in the day is less likely to be stored as fat. It takes about four hours for the food to be metabolized and for the nutrients, including energy, to enter the bloodstream.

This works like fuel for a furnace. If the furnace is banked for the night and a delivery of fuel arrives, it is stored for later use.

A heavy dinner eaten at 8 P.M. by a person who retires at 11 P.M. is like ordering fuel for a banked furnace. Coming up: wasted energy, and extra fat for the body's fat cells. And you know where that extra fuel and fat storage begins—and ends.

On the other hand, a heavy breakfast eaten at 7 A.M. by that same person is like ordering fuel for a furnace that needs all it can get.

Coming up: plenty of energy, and no storage of fat. And you know what that means—a slimmer you.

Morning and early afternoon food is current energy food. Late afternoon and evening food is future energy food. Future energy food is called fat.

This is one reason protein is less fattening. If you look at shorter time periods, as hour to hour instead of day to night, protein takes longer to digest and provides a smoother supply of energy for a few hours. On the other hand, carbohydrates—those sweets and starches—require less time to digest and come pouring into the bloodstream like a runaway freight train loaded with fuel. This can be far too much for the body's hourly needs, so the fat cells busy themselves and fat storage begins—and continues day by day.

Changing Eating Times Gradually

Shifting to an eating schedule earlier in the day is frequently a difficult procedure. We are creatures of habit. Change is threatening. We avoid, procrastinate, rationalize. We resist.

We are comfortable with retaining old, ingrained failure habits instead of learning and developing new, slenderizing success habits. We have learned to remain our own worst enemy. We stubbornly and foolishly refuse to become our own best friend.

Give yourself new instructions for changing your thinking and eating behavior—one day at a time.

If you have a disinclination to eat breakfast, then change gradually. Advance your first meal of the day earlier by one hour. Continue this schedule awhile. Then advance it earlier by another one or two hours. This gradual shift is easier to take. You are respecting your own habits. But, you are changing day by day. Once you are eating your first meal three or four hours earlier, you have now made room for two additional mini-meals.

Judith S., 35, had undesirable, fattening eating habits. Her five feet seven inches tipped the scales, almost over, at 215 pounds.

She ate from noon on. There were seldom special meal times. If there was a box of doughnuts around, it was a meal for her. A pint of

The Amazing Rule of Two

ice cream—another meal. She loved waffles, would often toast a whole box of eight frozen waffles and eat all of them at one sitting, drowned in syrup.

After work, she would meet her friends at their favorite bar. Six or eight shots of Scotch were par. She also enjoyed Margaritas.

Judith had to make some heavy decisions. Her heaviness was getting to be a social problem. She needed to think about how to resolve her problem. She realized her bar time was socializing time, but it was actually contributing to her inability to be a successful socializer.

How about camaraderie without drinks? She recalled that twenty years ago she would have a lot of fun with her friends without going to a bar. In those days, she drank milk. Why not move fun time from the bar to her house—and maybe even drink some milk (non-fat).

She decided to do this gradually. Two of her heavier friends were just as fond of playing gin as drinking it. They started a game. When others joined, it turned to poker. The hard drinks turned to soft diet (low-calorie) drinks or an occasional program-oriented milkshake or milk drink.

Then Judith was ready to begin the One-Day-At-A-Time Plan.

But she was not ready to eat breakfast. So she made a gradual shift. She carried a half grapefruit to work with her and two hard-boiled eggs and ate them at her 10 A.M. coffee break.

She arranged to have her lunch an hour later, at 2 P.M. and steered herself to the lunch counter instead of the bakery. She had a broiled hamburger steak with lettuce and tomatoes and a cup of black coffee. It tasted good. After work, playing cards, she counted her diet cola as a meal. Later, she had some cheddar cheese and a glass of skim milk.

Judith awoke the next morning feeling strange and wonderful. She never felt "alive" at 7 A.M. before. A more accurate word would be "dead." She stepped on the scale. She had lost three pounds during that one day.

That did it.

She ate breakfast.

During the next six days her weight dropped below 200—a loss of 16 pounds in one week!

Below is a record of the food she ate her second and third days on the One-Day Plan:

Wednesday	7 A.M.	½ grapefruit cottage cheese, low fat
	11 A.M.	celery, radishes, 1 oz. American cheese
	2 P.M.	6 oz. chicken beets, spinach
	6 P.M.	carrots, celery milk, non-fat
	10 P.M.	milk, non-fat
Thursday	7 A.M.	omelet, 2 eggs 1 oz. cheese 1 oz. ham, lean milk, non-fat
	1 P.M.	baked sole, lemon juice, green beans
	7 P.M.	red beans (10) and cabbage, lettuce and cucumber salad with oil and vinegar
	11 P.M.	celery milk, non-fat

It was an immense change for Judith, but she did it in small, gradual steps. Her immense weight continued to drop pound after pound, a fraction of a pound at a time, one day at a time.

The last time I saw her she was well on the way toward her goal of 120 pounds just by creating new eating habits—one small, gradual step at a time.

The Three-Day Plan—One Day At A Time

In order to make significant changes in your eating habits, you may want to go in easy stages.

If you do it in three stages over three days, for example, it is probably more accurate to call it a Three-Day Plan. But it still is one day at a time. And when you reach the next day, it is *that* day that counts.

The Amazing Rule of Two

There is another reason why three days are helpful. Some people require more time to become used to changes. They do not form new habits or shed old habits as quickly as others do.

These are the people who do not sleep soundly the first night or two in a hotel or some other strange place. Perhaps their bowels don't function normally when they travel. Home is their favorite place, because they know it better than any other place and strangeness makes them uncomfortable and tense. When they eat out, they are not adventuresome. They stick to the tried and the true. And the excess weight continues to stick to them.

These people need to apply the "Rule of Two" by merely splitting two items off their largest meals. Delay the salad and tea until two hours after lunch. Delay the cantaloupe and coffee until two hours after dinner.

This entails the least and the easiest change. Two or three days later the five meals can be made more definitive.

Other changes which my plan entails can also be more easily accepted after three days—or longer if necessary. One day can be commencing, but it does not clinch a decision. No matter how much you enjoyed the different way of eating and no matter how much better you feel, you may be a slow changer. Repeat. Repeat again.

You may wish to allow three days, like Lucille C. did. There were sweets she enjoyed. There were special eating times. She decided to change the sweets first, then add the two meals. She missed her pie à la mode on the first day, but she felt no great strain. She also missed her late show, TV cookies, and a mid-afternoon candy bar. She missed them less on the second day and even less on the third day.

On the fourth day, pie, ice cream, cookies, and candy never entered her mind. Here are Lucille's three days of menus.

First Day	Breakfast	2 scrambled eggs; ½ melon, coffee with skim milk
	Lunch	½ can tuna mixed with lettuce, celery, bell peppers; ½ grapefruit
	Dinner	sliced tomatoes (3), ½ cup cottage cheese, small steak, ½ cup spinach

Second Day	Breakfast	½ melon, coffee
	Lunch	1 hamburger pattie, lean, 1 apple, sliced cheese, coffee
	Dinner	1 chicken breast, ½ cup string beans; small green salad, diet dressing, coffee
Third Day	Breakfast	poached egg, ½ grapefruit, coffee
	Lunch	1 lamb chop, broiled, cup spinach, 4 strawberries, skim milk
	Dinner	small halibut steak, ½ cup carrots, ½ cup cabbage, coffee, diet jello

Lucille was proud of her five-pound weight loss. She decided to continue eating the way she was eating and to repeat the Three-Day Plan as often as necessary. It was effortless and satisfying.

A week later she decided to apply the "Rule of Two." She cut her portions and added a second breakfast and an afternoon tea to her "habits." This, too, required three days. She became fully accustomed to the new way. The new way then became her way—the slender, easy way.

Making a Meal out of Liquids

Adding two meals to your day is a must. But how and when you add them is a personal matter. I recommend adding them as early as possible in the day, but there my part ends and it becomes your decision. There are a number of factors that affect this decision making on your part.

The switch from sweets and starches to proteins has to be a gradual one, requiring a transitional period of a few days or longer. But don't drag your feet or procrastinate. Also, repeated or prolonged delays can lead to failure.

The switch from one to two breakfasts may also need a transitional period in which the interval between these two meals increases.

The switch from two to four mini-meals or from three to five mini-meals or even four to six mini-meals may require preparation. Shopping and menu planning are important so that the right foods are available in the right place at the right time.

There is another ingredient of the Schiff Plan which could be helpful at this point in deciding how to add two meals to your "agenda." You are asked to drink at least eight glasses of liquid.

Water is the best liquid. It is calorie free and should be a major part of your liquid intake. But decaffeinated coffee, weak tea, and diet soda may also be part of your liquid intake.

You can make a meal out of a liquid. A cup of coffee or a glass of tea is no meal. Neither is a bottle of soda. But a glass of skim milk can be a meal. And a glass of tomato juice can also be a meal.

A bowl of soup can be a meal—chicken broth, beef bouillon, or clam broth. Consommé Madrilene is a jellied soup that is served cold and makes a good summer meal.

Because we are accustomed to chewing during a meal, you may add a slice of cheese to this repast, or a few wedges of green pepper, stalks of celery, or carrot sticks, etc.

Any of the beverages listed among the recipes of the previous chapters can be a meal for you with the addition of a few accouterments such as cheese snacks, appetizers, or raw vegetables.

There are a number of canned liquid meals on the market that you may enjoy. These are similar to milkshakes and contain protein and nutritional supplements. Look for these in the special nutrition (dietetic) section of your supermarket. However, check content and total calories carefully.

A reminder: When you add meals, also add "kiks."

Select a liquid meal only if you enjoy what you are using for that liquid meal.

Enjoyment spells success on my plan more than it does on any diet. It is actually *your enjoyment* of that One Day that forms and perpetuates new habits, habits that add up to the new habit of being naturally slender—always.

The Pure Protein Drink As an Extra Meal

A few years ago a diet craze hit the United States, dwarfing all others that had gone before it. It consists of a liquid protein drink—available in health food stores, markets, and drug stores.

A person on this liquid protein diet abstains from food altogether and drinks the protein liquid four to six times a day.

Since this is approximately a 300-500 calorie regimen, free of sweets, starches, and fat, pounds drop away fast. But so can your health.

Many untoward side effects have been reported among people who have remained on this diet for several weeks. The body needs vitamins, minerals, and nutrients. It also needs some carbohydrates. The brain and nervous system are dependent on glucose, a product of the body's digestion of carbohydrates. Glucose is formed temporarily from vital protein when the body burns its own fat exclusively. This process should be limited to avoid unwanted effects on one's health.

Potassium is another important element that is missing. When the body becomes potassium-depleted, heart rhythm abnormalities can occur. It is believed that protein intake cannot be properly utilized when potassium and perhaps micro-amounts of other nutrients are not available.

I do *not* recommend that you use this liquid protein exclusively. Perhaps the only exception would be if you are extremely obese and this obese state is presenting an immediate and critical health problem. Even then, you should go on this liquid protein regimen only under the supervision of your physician or bariatrician (weight-control specialist).

However, there is absolutely no danger in using this liquid protein as a substitute for one meal or even two meals on the One-Day-At-A-Time Plan.

Its use *without* other meals is dangerous, especially over a prolonged period. However, its use as a supplement in conjunction *with* other meals is perfectly safe. It is safe because your other meals are supplying fat, carbohydrates, vitamins, potassium, and other minerals, plus the essential nutrients needed for your vital system to function properly.

You may enjoy the convenience of the liquid protein as a portable meal.

You may enjoy the taste of the liquid protein drink.

You may enjoy the way the liquid protein gives you a full feeling and how that feeling lasts until your next meal.

Again, "kiks" count. If you do not enjoy the liquid protein drink, it has no part to play on your program, as it will be "kikless" and unenjoyable.

On the other hand, you cannot enjoy what you have never experienced. So I propose using a so-called protein-supplemental drink as an option when planning additional low-calorie or mini-meals for your daily eating routine.

Use the liquid protein to add one or two meals daily to the One-Day-At-A-Time Plan. Use the liquid protein in this way as a supplement day after day if desired. See Chapter XII for maximum usage to accelerate weight loss. But if you intend to make all your meals liquid protein, see your physician before you begin.

A Word About Dietetic Foods

Recently one of my patients told me how she purchased some diet cookies to use with her favorite beverage as a meal. Halfway through them she read the label and noticed they had the same calorie value as regular cookies. She wondered why the manufacturer had a right to call them "low calorie."

There are guidelines for labeling the content of dietetic food products. Recently, the Federal Drug Administration did issue tentative regulations covering reduced calorie foods. Under these proposed guidelines, a food labeled "low calorie" would have to contain at least one third fewer calories than its counterpart food where calories have not been reduced.

But even with this improved labeling, what are you really eating? You are still eating sweets and starches. Maybe sorbitol has been substituted for the sugar—a sweetener that digests more slowly than sugar but which still has calories. Nothing has been substituted for the white flour.

So what change are you really making? As long as you are going to make a change, you may as well change effectively and you may as well change to something that tastes better, not worse. Cookies are cookies. They fatten easily. They are neither lasting pleasure nor are they nourishing. You pay a fat price. Buying cookies on a diet shelf instead of the regular cookie shelf is merely fooling yourself. Don't play foolish games.

Don't fool yourself. Feed yourself. Buy low-fat cottage cheese. Buy onions. Buy mushrooms. Chop the onions and mix them with the cottage cheese. Use the mushrooms to dip into the onioned cottage cheese. Now that's a lot better than a diet cookie. It is better in taste, better in nutrition, and costs no more. And, it is better in a weight-loss program.

Diet foods are prepared foods. Prepared foods are natural foods changed by processing methods. These processing methods do not add benefits to what nature has provided. They detract. Processing kills nutrients. It adds chemicals, preservatives, and colorants that do nothing beneficial for your body. You will be hungrier eating processed foods instead of natural produce because you are obtaining less nutrition per mouthful.

I am not condemning all diet foods. They are undoubtedly the answer for many people who must restrict or exclude salt or sugar. But are they the answer for you who are about to change your eating habits forever?

Do you want to live off a diet food shelf? Diet foods are temporary expedients. The Schiff Plan—as you know by now—is not a temporary expedient. It is a way of changing painlessly and permanently. Choose foods that delight the taste buds, the body, and the mind. Choose to lose.

Move away from that special diet department. It has "dead" food. Move over to the meat, fish, fresh frozen, and fresh produce departments. Here are "full-of-life" foods that are permitted in this program. These foods are nourishing and life supporting.

Also, I'm not condemning all canned or processed foods. What splendid meals and snacks some make! Where would we be without canned tuna, salmon, and herring? And what a convenience to have canned soups—the kind without flour (creamed) or sugar. Canned pineapple (drained of syrup) makes a good extra meal, as do canned pears or peaches. Always buy the water pack if available.

How to Experiment with Different Menu Plans Before Beginning the One-Day-At-A-Time Plan

Hopefully your book entitled "Me" is now ready.

Presumably you have taken care of the title page, made your first sugar monitoring entries, listed your favorite allowable foods, and recorded the foods that are now "off limits."

Imagine that you will begin the One-Day-At-A-Time program tomorrow. Use a page in your book to list the menu for that day.

The Amazing Rule of Two

Remember, you are really not starting tomorrow. What you are doing tomorrow is like a "dry run." List a transition type of day. Make gradual changes. Don't go all the way on dumping sweets and starches, just part of the way.

Don't go all the way, cutting the portions in half. Don't go all the way, applying the Rule of Two. Add only one meal. Patience. Time. Easy does it. Don't go all the way with eliminating disallowed foods. Permit a glass of beer or potatoes or a couple of slices of bread.

Write down your menu ahead of time in your book. Use a left-hand page. Then keep your book open. Check the menu as you proceed through the day, recording any additional foods that you eat that are not on the menu. Underscore these additions. Then immediately write on the opposite page about the circumstances that led to your consuming the added foods. These might be, "Offered to me and I could not refuse."

Or:

"Felt angry. Need to eat."

"Was turned down. Ate a sweet."

"Feel bored, depressed, lonely."

"Annoyed by the children."

"Nothing else to do."

"There it was in front of me."

"She begged me to try it."

"I love ice cream so much."

What are some of your special circumstances?

These are the kinds of pressures and rationalizations we erroneously translate into appetite (false hunger). These errors of translation leave their fatty mark on us.

There is a joke we doctors hear repeatedly: When an architect makes a mistake, he can grow ivy over it, but when a doctor makes a mistake, he can only bury it. Well, you have a problem, too, in hiding your mistaken hunger. It bulges here and protrudes there for all to see. And, your mirror doesn't lie to you.

To correct your false hunger (appetite), you need to monitor yourself—your thoughts and feelings—when you eat. The correct "translations" then take place automatically without any illogical, self-deceiving willpower or trying. The fatty marks fade away and disappear. The slender you gradually appears.

What better time to start than now when you are about to

experiment with different menu plans, prior to beginning the One-Day-At-A-Time Plan?

For some the monitoring is a restrained procedure. The feelings are subtle. For others, it is like watching an electric storm, full of the fury of thunder and lightning. The feelings cry out.

That is the way it was for Gladys F., 39, a teacher, all 200 pounds of her. She wrote the following in her book when beginning to monitor herself:

It's four in the morning and unless I write or do something to help myself, I am going to burst. I am under so much pressure. I don't know if I can take it, and eating won't help. It will just add one more thing to hurt about. The last couple of days have really been tough.

My cleaning lady didn't come, so I had to spend Saturday housecleaning. My back always rebels at bending over and doing floors. So I have a clean house, but my floors are dirty.

The next day we went to my husband's friends' house to watch the football games. The woman served only fattening foods. I was lucky enough to anticipate the problem and ate beforehand. But still, when she served pizza for dinner, how could I not eat it? She put a bowl of donuts in front of me and left it there for two hours! But I was not nice and ate some of them.

Also, my husband's lack of consideration aggravated me. I felt hurt and angry because he spent several hours in front of the TV while I had to keep our hyperactive five-year-old happy in someone else's house. Although I had brought toys for him, that did not do the trick.

I felt ragged when I went home. Because of him and the socially acceptable food which I was not allowed to eat, I ate more pizza to soothe my nerves.

Then today, Monday, everything seemed to go wrong. I have been trying to get a permanent teacher's contract, but last week I unfortunately reached the school system's maximum weight. Now I find I am on a list for contracts, but I'm 23rd in line. That means no contract this year. I will have all the responsibilities of a regular teacher, but I'll be paid $3000 less a year than my academic background and teaching experience entitle me to. We are presently in a financial bind and need the extra money. I told my husband that it sure makes me want to eat something bad. He said, "No, stick to your plan. You are on the plan for you and not for the Board of Education." I ate a huge salad with ice tea and didn't turn to food for consolation. Still another problem, my principal called a special meeting after school on Wednesday and gave us only 48 hours notice. This is the same day I take my little boy to religion class and there is no one I can ask to take him. I won't tell you what that made me eat.

Sounds like enough, right—no, not yet. Today I had a run in with a student who refused to put away outside work in my class. I had asked him to cooperate several times, but he didn't. When I called him on it, he refused to cooperate and caused an unnecessary scene in front of the entire class. I'll have to seek the help of his counselor to straighten him out or suspend him.

So, that's why I'm awake at 4 A.M. feeling both angry at the damn school system and sorry for myself. I have about 50 pounds to lose, yet I have such a promiscuous appetite.

Another thing is bothering me—premenstrual tension for which I know of no cure. I'm feeling very emotional and vulnerable. I need support and there is no one to help me. Now I know how an alcoholic must think and feel. Alone and trapped by your own inadequacies.

This past weekend and today have just about convinced me I need to help myself to get me over the hump of dealing with all the mess I am in at one time.

"Gladys, help yourself by programming and reprogramming ODAAT (one day at a time)—unlearn, relearn, unthink, rethink, untrain, retrain, undo, redo—peel away the layers of mental fat—negative and unwanted thoughts, emotions, attitudes, habits, etc. You never get over or under the hump (mental road blocks you have developed) unless you PAL (permit, allow, let), make, cause, do—to lead yourself through the mounds of garbage and shovel it away, layer by layer, ODAAT. Don't give yourself the short end of the deal and deal yourself from the bottom of the deck—don't allow the cards to control you—a fool's game. Don't deal with the whole mess at one time (you made it). Just as it required a long time to build the mess (negative situations), it requires time and patience to clear it away day by day; also to build the correct or desirable situations (experiences, events). Learn to love yourself."

Seven weeks later and 24 pounds lighter Gladys F. wrote:

Things (I, me) have definitely improved. The lady who told me I would not get a work contract was wrong! Boy, am I happy! I ironed out all the other problems as well WITHOUT RESORTING TO THE COMFORT AND SECURITY OF A TUMMY FULL OF CARBOHYDRATES. Bravo for me! It's getting easier and easier to handle everyday problems and aggravations day-by-day without eating them away. In fact, I made cupcakes for my son and am very proud that they remained until they went stale, because I did not eat them.

I am finding I'm becoming so used to the food on the program that the No No's don't bother me anymore. In fact, sometimes in the cafeteria I look at the "glop" they serve and wonder how I could have ever eaten that stuff! I head for the fresh salad bar and have become an alfalfa sprout nut! Who would have ever thought it? I never ate anything green until I was 30 years old!

Begin your adventure in self-exploration. You may be amazed how it helps the false hunger (appetite) and real pounds to disappear. And you may be amazed how it allows the true hunger and alluringly slender you to appear.   Truly a miracle.

VIII

WHAT TO DO WHEN YOU ARE NOT ON THE PLAN TO KEEP THE POUNDS COMING OFF

Excess poundage is an abnormality. Which means it *is not* the normal, healthy state of the body. Other abnormalities are usually called diseases or illnesses or malfunctioning. Excess poundage gets away with murder, yet it is not called a disease. But it is. It represents *dis-ease*. It also represents an abnormal body.

Doctors are finding that more and more diseases of the body are caused by negative and undesirable attitudes, distressed feelings, and disturbed emotions. For example—colds, upset stomach, intestinal problems, ulcers, skin rashes, muscular and joint disorders, even cancer. Statistically, a large percentage of medical problems are psychosomatic in origin, which also means that excess poundage *is not* the normal, healthy state of the mind.

Recently, Professor Claus Bahnson, a psychiatrist at Philadelphia's Thomas Jefferson University, stated in a newspaper interview that in five or ten years psychological screening will be able to predict up to 70 percent of cancer cases.

For instance, Dr. Bahnson says that women who have lived in a state of conflict with their mothers, who do not accept their role as women, and who resent sex, seem to be especially susceptible to cancer.

He describes the typical cancer patient as a person who was emotionally upset as a child, but kept unpleasant experiences hidden, and now finds it difficult to express anger or hurt.

The monitoring, understanding, and control of thoughts, emotions, feelings and attitudes are helping to handle stress and many other disease-causing factors.

They are also helping to cure obesity. *In fact, they are the most important aspects in the control and eventually the complete eradication of obesity!*

They are also significant keys to achieving permanent and gratifying weight loss!

Is this food for thought? I hope so.

My patients and I know this to be so. You will know this to be so by the time you finish reading this book. Because in this chapter I am going to give you ways to "spy" on yourself that may save your life!

You do not have to do this on the One-Day-At-A-Time Plan, but it will help. You *do* have to do this on the days before and after the One-Day Plan.

That means today—now!

Today counts the most. It is the most important day of your life. The past cannot be changed. The future cannot be reached. Today is here and now. It is the first day of the rest of your life.

"Reaching my desired weight is no longer the only goal for me," states Helen M., 62. "It is the one day at a time—thinking, eating, understanding, daily living, and achieving."

Well stated, Helen. We all have a desired weight goal. But if we attach that weight to a date, it adds to frustration. Frustration leads to false hunger. Appetite leads to fat-dom.

We must end frustration. Moreover, we must end all unwanted emotions and attitudes that create false hunger (appetite).

Unwanted emotions and negative attitudes are easily ended. It is a simple two-step procedure:
1. Identify.
2. Understand.

How to Identify Fattening Thoughts

Most of us have an easy time telling others about our problems. All we seem to need is a willing ear and out they pour. Let it flow.

This makes us feel better. Talking about them seems to be good for us. In fact, talking about our problems is the main thrust of psychotherapy. What is there to talking about problems that seems to relieve them? Well, in talking about them you are identifying them. And you are also helping to understand them and yourself.

Bartenders are therapists. Their therapy is not the liquor they serve; it is their attentiveness to their customers' problems. Beauticians are therapists. Yes, their cosmetic skills help, but listening to their clients' problems can help much more.

What to Do When You Are Not on the Plan

I recently had a beautician as a patient. She would tell me about patients who were her clients. At one time she had six clients who were either my patients or were using one of my previous books and telling her about their emotional problems and attitudes. I admire her descriptions:

"Joy F. has been coming to me for years. She was about 100 pounds overweight. When I gave her a shampoo it was difficult to lean over and reach around her. She told me a few weeks ago she had started your program. She does not count calories. She is off junk food. She says she does not feel she is on a diet; she is just eating sensibly and straightening out her emotional problems.

"Well, you should see her today. She comes into the shop looking like a young, attractive woman. She feels great. She does not complain about her aching joints. She used to bring a hamburger on a bun, french fries, coke, potato chips, and cake. Now when she comes for a shampoo, permanent, and styling, she brings a few chicken legs and black coffee.

"When I ask her the secret of her new exuberance, she just says she is getting her life together. She used to be grumpy and complaining. Now she's all smiles and instead of 50-cent tips she now leaves 2-dollar tips!"

What was Joy's secret? I happen to know. It was writing about her thoughts and problems as though she were talking to a psychiatrist. She wrote, wrote, and wrote. She was not one to talk to a beautician; neither did she want to go for therapy to a psychiatrist or psychologist. She was confident she could identify and understand herself—by herself.

It is not hard to do, day by day. It is really easy and fun.

The book called "ME" is a special kind of story, kept by you for you. Many of my patients gave me theirs—and some have given me permission to quote from their books in the book you now have in your hands. I thank them for sharing so that others may benefit.

I have seen men and women relate their innermost thoughts in black and white. Some are deeply soul-touching. Some are X-rated. Some are lightning and thunder.

These thoughts are fattening. They are the reasons for false hunger. Once they are recorded they become as thin as the paper they are written on. Recording them on paper is a way of capturing them. Capturing them is a way of identifying and understanding them. Once identified and understood, they are neutralized. Then those thoughts are no longer able to control you. You have captured them. You control them. It is like defusing a bomb.

Can you imagine a man weighing 317 pounds? That is a lot of meat even on a six-foot frame. Jerry W., 37, was overweight all his life. No diet or medication ever succeeded for him. And he never succeeded. I first saw him in December, 1975. The last time I saw him was in October, 1976. In those ten months he lost 76 pounds effortlessly and was still losing.

Jerry attributed his success to the monitoring of his own feelings and recording them on paper. But let Jerry tell you himself as he writes to lose more weight:

"I have been to several doctors and have been on several programs in the past for my weight problem. Many times I was treated with medication alone but given no psychological help. I knew I had a long way to go to lose all the weight and I would have to proceed slowly—there was much to be done.

"I couldn't handle my emotional problems, eating binges and compulsive eating. Even though I was aware of my negative behavior and attitudes I was powerless to stop it—like a train going down the track, and not being able to apply the brake.

"I would find lots of excuses and would eat without any control—five slices of bread each meal, ice cream, candy bars, etc. I know my problem is emotional; my thoughts trigger the need for a release to let out pent up steam. I turned to food as a safety valve.

"It gives me an immediate blockage of thoughts and feelings and numbs me for awhile. Of course this is all coupled with being unemployed, lying about the house and feeling sorry for myself. I think if I could straighten out my thinking and could become productive in society and for myself, I would have a lot to contribute and pour out of myself. Unfortunately, I have no constructive channels for release. All this energy is turned inward toward destructive abuse against myself and is wasted.

"I noticed when I was engaged in a satisfying job I really had no craving to eat or run to food. In the absence of a satisfying occupation the energy is turned inward, destructively. This accounts for a great deal of my problem. As soon as I awaken in the morning I feel defeated.

"We just had a baby and I have to find a job. It's hard to motivate myself as I feel very conscious about this weight. I want to be and feel happy. I'll never be this age again so I want to enjoy it now.

What to Do When You Are Not on the Plan

"During the period from January, 1976, until now I have studied my lecture notes and have repeated this material over and over. I think this has helped me 'screw my head around.' I am thinking about and understanding many things I had failed to do in the past.

"Perhaps the greatest realization for me—learning to change my mind and lifestyle—has helped me to control my intake of food.

"The writing, reading, and meditating techniques plus the other instructions have helped me to understand myself. I'm thinking more clearly and learning to do one day at a time! Being in control of food intake was a gradual process; however, it never seemed to me that I was on a diet at any time.

"I follow the Food Guide—this is a very easy way to go compared to some of the rigid diets of the past.

"Actually, I diet about one day a month when I cut back drastically on quantity of food. I suppose eating sensibly and eliminating all the junk foods, beer and pretzels, alcohol, candy, bread and other No-No's has made it easy for me to continue losing weight gradually. I've learned—I now eat to live.

"But I'm in no hurry and the routine of 'dieting' once a month now, the good eating principles, plus your help in thought, attitude and emotional behavior, leads me to believe that I will reach my desired weight in due time. I am working steady the past seven months and have other interests to occupy my leisure time. This helps a lot. I think I'm a happier person now."

Jerry sounds like his own analyst, doesn't he? That's because he is. And so are the thousands of others who have become permanently slender by programming only one day at a time, and maybe not for many repeats.

What thoughts do you have and watch for? Which thoughts are negative, ego-sapping, and fattening?

Well, here are a few of the more common ones "unearthed" by my self-analyzing patients:

My boring job (exhausting, tenuous, dangerous, demanding, nerve wracking)

My inability to get a job (or make sales, meet people, get clients, etc.)

My irritating boss (supervisor, co-worker, mate, neighbor, in-laws, etc.)

My sexually unresponsive mate (or cheating, bored, gambling, drinking)

My fear of meeting new people (of small rooms, of elevators, of high places, of crowds, of being alone, of the dark, of driving, of success, etc.)

My worry about electric storms (earthquakes, tornadoes, floods, etc.)

My inability to attract a love partner (or have an orgasm, erection, or sensuous thought)

My concern about the children (getting sick, leaving home, becoming pregnant, getting into trouble)

My feelings about my own worthlessness (unattractiveness, lack of skills, obesity, etc.)

My despondency (futility, pessimism, disappointment, frustration, melancholy, depression, mourning, etc.)

My anger (hate, jealousy, resentment, hostility, etc.) toward —————.

These comprise perhaps 90 percent of the many fattening thoughts.

They are fattening because they are mentally painful to have, so we take our mind off them by eating and overeating—anything.

You could be given the best diet in the whole world, with every detail spelled out for you morning to night, day after day, month after month. *If* you continue to have these negative, unwanted, confused thoughts, you will discontinue the diet—eventually.

Diets are useless unless these thoughts are identified and "handled." It is not totally accurate to say that in addition to a physical plan you need to go on a mental plan too, although I sometimes use this expression. It is not accurate because you do not deprive yourself of the fattening thoughts. You just don't allow these old, unhappy, fattening thoughts to prevail any more because you have decided to replace them with new, happy, slenderizing thoughts.

In order to make this decision, you must decide NOW—today. Then, do!

Substitute or switch thoughts—and emotions. Look at and think about the brighter aspects of life. Thus, you will cultivate new and enlightened attitudes toward life. Then—YOU light up *your* life.

Just as we substitute proteins for sweets, starches, and fat on the physical level, we substitute creative, healthful, positive thoughts for destructive, health-sapping, negative thoughts on the mental level. By this process of substituting or switching on the physical and mental levels, we substitute a slender person for an overweight person.

It seems like a long way off. But it is much closer than you think.

Monitoring Fattening Thoughts One Day At A Time

So many overweight people consider the task so immense and the goal so unreachable that they give up almost before they start.

Jerry's extra 100 pounds was a formidable project. It was like deciding to go on a ten-mile hike in a blinding snowstorm with the snow already two feet deep.

But Jerry went one day at a time. When you go on such a hike one pace at a time, often, before you realize, the snow stops falling and you soon reach a place where little or no snow has fallen.

Instead of getting harder and harder, it becomes easier and easier, one day at a time.

Instead of looking at your final weight goal, do the programming (self-instructing) one day at a time.

Instead of continuing to wallow in emotional garbage—monitor it, observe it, identify it, understand it, then discard it forever.

Each day does indeed bring you closer to your weight goal. And each day you monitor your thoughts and emotions does indeed bring you closer to understanding yourself, accepting yourself, and loving yourself.

But today is *the* day. Decide to take a look at yourself today. Not in the full-length mirror you used earlier in this book, but in the mirror of your mind—your thoughts, perceptions, and imagination. *Learn to see with the "mind's eye." Instruct yourself.*

Open the book called "ME." Sit quietly. Relax. Ponder. Think.

What do you know about your emotions that blare forth like the sound of a thousand trumpets?

A person who works in a cymbal factory grows used to the sound of clatter and clang. Ask him if it's noisy at work and he'll probably shrug his shoulders and say, "No more than in other jobs." You are used to those thousand trumpets in your mind which you translate as "appetite bells." You are used to worry, anxiety, self-pity, or whatever dark, unhappy, fattening thoughts you have. You no longer hear the piper you are dancing to.

Unless you stop, look, and listen. . . .

Just today. Just right now. Stop, look, and listen.

With your book called "ME" open to a blank page and with pen or pencil in hand, be quiet and observe what you begin to think about. . . .

There! See? Quick! Write it down.

Everybody's thoughts are different. Your thoughts may have had absolutely nothing to do with the most common fattening thoughts I enumerated before (pages 145–6). It does not mean that you have the wrong thoughts. If you have been at ease about these processes, you have gone right to the target—slenderizing thoughts. On the other hand, you may have been protecting your privacy from yourself. Off target—fattening thoughts.

There is no shame or guilt in this process. You are you. You have the right to be the way you are. You are the best friend you have. You can "level" with yourself. Level and be understanding. Level and be friendly. Level and be slender.

"Running off at the mind" is the way Mrs. Arlene C., 48, called this process. She was not ashamed to share her monitoring with me and others:

"I'm afraid I'll fail—not measure up (to what?) to my expectations? (which?) to be really great at anything I do.

"There have been many things I've never attempted, (chicken-shit) so many fears. (what fears?)

"Change—for one—and I don't take many risks. How terrible—I've let so much go by. *Risk* could mean *change* and change can be good. Why am I afraid of change? Because I don't know what it will bring. It's the unknown to me. Sometimes I have held on to situations, people, (God knows what else) painful situations. (Wow! Also my fat!) Good God! I'm holding on to that, too.

"And what could I lose—nothing but fat. What else could I lose? BOREDOM—I'll do more! Hey! This is getting exciting!

"Why do I have to be perfect at everything? Can't I just enjoy doing something without competing? Good Lord! *Perfection* to me deals with *competing*. My God! Competing with my sisters—always competing—for

Daddy's attention or recognition. He never even mentioned my name. I can't ever remember him calling my name—and if you are not called by name then you simply don't exist, do you? Is that why I have to be perfect? So that someone will recognize that I exist?

"Well—I damn well *do* exist, *I* know I do!"

These are inner thoughts. These are revealing. And once they reveal you to yourself, you are halfway home. You have identified the "black thoughts," the negative, confused, and depressing thoughts.

Just the way you are more in control of your food intake when you identify those two white substances as the nutritional culprits, you are more in control of your thoughts when you recognize the "black thoughts" which are the psychological (emotional) culprits. And these are "fattening thoughts."

Monitoring Techniques That Help Trap "Black Thoughts"

"Black thoughts" need light. When you throw light on "black thoughts," they change. They lighten. You lighten.

But some days it is not easy to monitor. You are too busy, too involved, too caught up in the emotional storms. How can you observe your thoughts when your spouse is three hours late? How can you observe your thoughts when your son has wrecked the car? How can you observe your thoughts when your boss has passed you by and given the promotion to someone else?

Even Arlene, whose candid self-analysis you just read, had days when she could not step out of herself long enough to observe herself. "I seem to be avoiding my feelings today. Maybe yesterday and today have been just too tough."

But just by writing that reason for not writing, she began to write more:

"Oh yes, I do remember something. I used to make promises that I had no intention of fulfilling. No one could fulfill the kind of promises I would make."

Coming up: new insight. New insight spells self-enlightenment. Self-enlightenment dispels "black thoughts." And once these thoughts are dispelled and replaced with "lighter" thoughts, the desire to eat when you are really not hungry vanishes. You become like any other slender person. You become a lighter person—both physically and mentally.

Keep "ME" nearby, preferably opened to a blank page and with a pencil or ballpoint pen handy and ready to go. An open book invites you to be an open book. It will encourage you at least to begin to write. Once you begin you trigger a flow of words, emotions, and thoughts. When the flow begins, write as fast as you can. If it stops, read what you have written, then new thoughts will soon begin to flow. Again, capture them.

Some people find it easier to write if they know it will be read. You can pick a family member or close friend and let that person "in" on the process. Or you can pick me. I guarantee I will read whatever you send to me. I may even write to you. If it is helpful for you to have someone at the other end of your writing, write in letter fashion. If it is easy to write to yourself, then write in diary fashion. But do write. Write now!

Arlene would let her writing go. Then one day when that open book and the clean white pages beckoned to her, she wrote:

"Consistency. Wow! Now there is something that has always bothered me. I just wasn't consistent about anything. I did not and still do not know how—but I am beginning to see that you must do it, do it, do it every day. That is why I am doing this. I can. I will. I must. It is like saving my life. The suffering I have endured because of my thinking and eating habits is . . . I don't know a word for it . . . excruciating. No, that's not word enough. But now I will be consistent. I will write. I will persist. I will grow from IT as a person and grow smaller as a body. That's the plan, and writing is part of it."

Need I say more?

A Transformation Takes Place in Your Record of Thought Monitoring

Lightening of the body comes one pound at a time, one day at a time. But enlightenment of the mind can come suddenly—like lightning. Once lightning strikes, you no longer have to pay any

What to Do When You Are Not on the Plan

attention to the lightening. You lighten automatically—like air coming out of a balloon once the string is untied.

Your mental knots are keeping the fat in you. Untie them by writing and slender down to normal without a diet per se.

Are you beginning to read me? Then let me read you. Write. And watch the lightning strike and the lightening begin. You will know when lightning strikes. There may be no clap of thunder, but you will feel like clapping.

Would you like to see Arlene's lightning?

"I feel great lately; I seem to be more motivated. That's important to me. I want to make beautiful things for myself. Also, I thought about taking discothèque dancing when I lose another ten pounds.

"Why do I feel I must wait? Why don't I start now? That's a great *idea*. NOW. That's what it's all about. Following through. Doing. Doing now and not waiting. I think I've spent my life waiting. My God! There's only one time. And it's now. There is only one day and it is today. One year—now.

"NOW. NOW. NOW!"

That's what I call lightning. It was easy for Arlene from then on. She started her discothèque dancing. She began living the life of a slender, lighter person. And she became one. It was a breakthrough, a miracle.

You will have a breakthrough, too.

I see "breakthrough" in my office *every day*. People shed their armor, their false security—and their weight.

The patient disrobes for a doctor's examination. But frequently, more than clothes come off:

"Your seeing me, knowing and understanding," writes one patient, "made me ever so vulnerable. It was like being nude and looked at—And I mean nude inside."

Fat is armor. It protects the bruised and insecure feelings that you have bottled up inside. As long as you have and hold onto those feelings, you will need the fat. Eliminate the unwanted feelings and black thoughts by identifying and understanding them—and you no longer need the fatty armor.

Which means you no longer need to do what these people are doing:

A 60-year-old woman stops in the fudge shop and finishes the pound before returning home.

A teenage boy washes "Twinkies" down with a coke—every few hours.

A young man spends an hour at a bar on the way home from work downing beer and pretzels.

A housewife serves herself first and begins eating before the others are served, winding up having seconds and thirds.

A lawyer meets with his clients for breakfast, lunch, and dinner, always at the finest restaurants, going for "the works" and picking up the tab.

Everyone has his or her own way of feeding the armor, strengthening the protection around those private idiosyncracies by increasing the layers of physical and mental fat:

(Why should anyone know my husband no longer comes to my bed?)

(Why should anyone know I'm afraid to kiss a girl?)

(Why should anyone know I hate my parents?)

(Why should anyone know I've been bored to death all day?)

(Why should anyone know I've lost seven of my last eight cases?)

Each one of these five parenthetical inner situations can be paired with a specific person among the five described above. Can you pair the correct situation to the specific person? Obviously, the first person, the 60-year-old fudge eater, is paired with the first situation, the empty bed. The second person with the second situation, etc.

How do you pierce the armor? How do you eliminate the false security—fat? By daily writing. By daily self-understanding. By daily thinking, programming—and doing.

You Begin to Lose Those Unwanted Pounds When You Pierce the Mental Armor

Marilyn J., 32, did not lose weight on the One-Day-At-A-Time Plan. She also did not write. I connected the two, and I was correct. But, confronted with this, Marilyn still demurred. She would not say why.

Two weeks after I had seen her for the first time the scale still pointed to 179 pounds.

"At least I did not gain" was her weak defense.

What to Do When You Are Not on the Plan

Few people resist my urging to write as strongly as Marilyn resisted, which made me prescribe "strong medicine."

"Don't see the receptionist for another appointment," I said as she prepared to leave.

"Won't you see me again?"

"Yes, of course I'll see you, but you have to write for an appointment. You know what I mean."

In a week I received a request for an appointment and enclosed was the following:

"Well, here I am doing what I dreaded the most, writing and thinking. I can see now that there is no way to avoid this. I guess eating habits are established early in life. And this is the part of my life I didn't want to think about, my past (this is a very tragic and unhappy part of my life). I've tried for many years to forget it. This is where the problem began.

"My parents were alcoholics. I had three brothers, one older and two younger. There was no excuse for the way we lived. I used to pray that someone would turn them over to the authorities, but no one ever did. Where were all the humanitarians then? We lived in a better than average section of town, in Santa Monica, north of Montana. They drove a Cadillac. My father had tailor-made suits and imported shoes. They belonged to the country club. But all four of us kids were living in the worst kind of hell. The same thing every day—it never changed. They'd come home at 9:00 P.M. every night, bringing with them one saucy dog (from Von's Market) for each one of us kids. Never more than one, never anything different, always a saucy dog. As for my father, he ate the biggest, thickest steaks you ever saw. Oh yes, we mustn't forget her cats (she had about 25 of them), and she'd have a large grocery bag of Skippy's cat food for them. As a matter of fact, that's all there ever was in the cabinets; cat food and brandy bottles. Well, all four of us kids were very thin. We were very close as we had no one else. I felt the sorriest for my youngest brother. I guess being the youngest, he got the worst of it.

"The stage was already set for something to happen. My oldest brother started dipping into the brandy bottles and to smoke. My middle brother started to retreat from people in embarrassment. My youngest brother started to mess in his pants and to stammer and stutter. The only thing I could do was to run as fast and as far as I could. The final result: My youngest brother went completely insane and had to be locked up in a state mental hospital (he still isn't right to this day). My middle brother is so weird it's impossible to get along with him. He's so immaculate and precise, you all but have to make an appointment to see him. My oldest brother died last year of a heroin overdose. He was only 33 years old. I ran away, met and married my first husband when I turned 16."

Marilyn was writing about the very heart of her problem. It went way back to her childhood. Somehow, when we take pen in hand, it hits the target. She began to lose steadily after that. In less than six months she had shed 61 pounds and was a svelte 126 pounds. Bullseye!

You may not have a scarred past or a desperate present. But you do have something. Put it on paper and stop putting it in your mouth and on your body.

You start to lose weight. It drops off without any conscious regulating. You just find that eating correctly is right for you—your way, every day, every One Day.

How the Power of Thought Shapes Our Ends

Thoughts, attitudes, emotions and feelings are more important than you realize.

Thoughts are like your private world. You think because they are never heard, seen, or communicated to others, they are hidden in a safe place. No way. They eventually surface in one form or another, no matter how secretive you are.

Science is now studying the energy of thoughts. It is found to be a very real energy that can be photographed and measured on various meters. It affects the environment, external and internal.

This study is relatively new. It is called Psychotronics. In one of the few popular books* on this new science, Dr. Robert B. Stone of Honolulu tells how to focus this energy of consciousness or thought to make changes in your life as if by magic, including the overcoming of financial obstacles, improving health, and making wishes come true.

In writing as I have asked you to do, you are using this energy. Writing focuses the energy of consciousness, flushes out fears and resentments; also other imbalancing thoughts, feelings, emotions and

---

*"The Magic of Psychotronic Power," Parker Publishing Co., Inc., West Nyack, N.Y., 1978

What to Do When You Are Not on the Plan

attitudes. It restores perfect mental balance. It eliminates dis-ease. And, not so incidentally, it slenderizes.

With perfect mental equilibrium, your physical equilibrium improves, too. Mental composure composes the body as it decomposes the excess fat.

Thought has the power to shape our ends, in the spiritual, psychological (emotional), social—and, in the physical sense. Extra pounds on the buttocks, arms, legs, hips, thighs, abdomen, and other locations mean extraneous, dark thoughts on the mind. These thoughts need to be captured by you, identified and understood. Writing is an easy, inexpensive, quick and gratifying way to do this. It makes the One-Day-At-A-Time Plan work better than any thirty- or sixty-day diet—only if *you* work day by day.

The choice is yours.

If you choose to join the ranks of the forever slender by agreeing now with yourself to write, you are going to make and see some "magic" take place in your life. You will amaze yourself. The results will be miraculous!

How much time do you think it took between this page in Beryl G.'s book called "ME" and the next one that follows it?

"While we're on the subject of *hurts*, I recall another incident that only happened a few months ago.

"My husband needed some work done on one of his trucks. He told the mechanic when he was finished with the truck to just come on by the house and drop the truck keys off with his wife. When he was finished he came by the house and gave me the truck keys.

"The next day when my husband came home he told me the mechanic had congratulated him about my pregnancy!

"That really embarrassed me and I know it must have embarrassed my husband too."

Here is another page from Beryl's "ME."

"I just returned from the market. I got such a laugh out of what happened that I just had to write about it.

"I was just taking a cart out and I turned around and right behind me was my *sister-in-law*. Well, naturally I immediately said, "Hi." She gave me a real strange look and finally said "Hello." She said *she did not even recognize me*.

"I had just seen them around the end of March and now it is only May.

"Also, I ran into another couple of people who have known me for years. They hadn't seen me in quite some time, as a matter of fact, since I started on this program.

"*Well, neither of these two people recognized me*—they stated very plainly that they wouldn't have if I had not spoken to them first."

The answer is seven months. Seven months for Beryl to go from 180 to 120 pounds. And from

these measurements:		to these:
Bust	37	34¾
Waist	34	27½
Hips	42	34¾
Thighs	26	20½

In her book "ME," Beryl hardly ever wrote about eating. She did write about her husband taking her to nicer restaurants where she could get high-protein meals instead of something junky like hot dogs or pizza or other junk food.

She did write about how she cooked with only the most nourishing ingredients and how her family enjoyed her cooking more.

But Beryl was not "diet" conscious.

She was "self" conscious. *She was "program" or "plan" conscious.*

So it is with the One-Day-At-A-Time program. It does involve switching foods, but once the switch has taken place, the idea of dieting dims and vanishes, along with your excess pounds.

You remain conscious, not of food you are not eating, but of thoughts you are not thinking. You celebrate the happy thoughts that replace the gloomy ones. You celebrate a happier and slimmer you.

You gain in mental "kiks" just as you are gaining in eating "kiks." And your gain is your body's loss.

In the next chapter we are going to experience simple ways to instruct the mind to automatically drop and dismiss the unwanted thoughts that "bug" us and cause unneeded eating, and to substitute wanted (happy), slenderizing thoughts in their place.

You could call it meditation, self-hypnotism, autoconditioning, re-education—and you would be basically correct.

I call it instructing the mind, because that is what it accomplishes.

It instructs the mind that there is a better way, and it helps the mind to be there and to "latch onto" these new, uplifting, slenderizing instructions.

It helps the mind develop awareness. It helps change your conscious and subconscious state of mind. And it helps eliminate those unwanted pounds forever.

You will get a "kik" out of the next chapter.

Then in the subsequent chapters, you will receive more information on how to derive more "kiks" out of food, how to control your weight loss—speed it up or slow it down—and how to remain slender without ever dieting again.

IX

MENTAL INSTRUCTIONS THAT END FAULTY EATING AND THINKING HABITS PRACTICALLY OVERNIGHT

Endless experience has proven, beyond a shadow of a doubt, that diets per se lead to eventual failure for the majority of dieters. Few diets, if any, include a procedure such as the one in which I am about to instruct you. Yet it is essential for meaningful and permanent success.

You have learned to eat the way you have been eating. It is the wrong way. It is killing you before your time, meanwhile robbing you of life's pleasures. Self-destruction is a foolish game.

You need to learn another way. But learning in the standard method of repetition takes longer than one day. You have to substitute eggs for danish, chopped steak for spaghetti, and cheese for apple pie again and again.

The more you enjoy the switch, the more likely you will repeat. Then the learning process will be insured. Self-preservation is a sensible game.

But as the old saying goes, "There's many a slip between the cup and the lip." And, there's many a slip between the mind and the mouth. *Think before, while eating, after you eat. Have some food, but first, have some thoughts.*

The procedure I am about to explain to you is a way of giving the mind immediate instructions and learning. It is hard to believe, *but instant learning is possible.*

The primary ingredients for learning are:
1. Relaxation
2. Imagination
3. Repetition

Learning is conditioning, programming, self-instructing. It is absorbing, then fixing new thoughts and ideas in your mind. It is disconnecting old, negative unwanted ideas, habits, emotions, and attitudes. It is connecting new, positive, desirable eating and thinking patterns.

You must learn to change your mind day by day in order to change your eating habits and control your weight permanently. The pathway to your body is through your mind.

This is done by learning in a relaxed state. This is not new. At one time sleep learning was quite popular. People who wanted to learn a foreign language would turn on an automatically repeating tape next to their bed and when they awoke in the morning they discovered that much of the vocabulary that was on that tape was now familiar to them.

Today, hypnotism and self-hypnotism are being used to learn new habits quickly. These methods have generally had a poor reputation among educators who prefer to stick to the tried and true methods of drills, memorizing, and repetition.

Even though unwanted habits such as smoking and overeating can be controlled through relearning via hypnotism and self-hynotism, physicians, too, prefer the tried and true, more orthodox approaches.

Expectant mothers, though, are being taught to ease childbirth pains by mental instructions; dental surgeons are using these methods to anesthetize the gums prior to tooth extraction.

In Bulgaria, a system of learning has been developed called Suggestology. While the students relax on couches and listen to symphony music, the professor intones the foreign language vocabulary lesson for the day. When they leave the class, the students have paid little conscious attention to the professor, yet they have learned considerably more than a standard class.

There is a simple formula that makes instant learning possible: relaxation + visualization (imagination) = learning. Repetition, day by day, insures the formula's success.

If you *relax* and *visualize* the way you want to eat and think, you automatically eat and think that way. You'll be that kind of a person. And you'll become a slimmer person.

No sweets and very little flour may be a difficult path for you right now, even for one day. But were you to relax and visualize yourself deriving "kiks" out of the protein foods instead of sweets and starches, you would take a giant step toward reaching your desired weight by being that kind of person. You will be a slimmer person with lots of "kiks."

And if you were to relax, visualize, and think about yourself, about your own pleasures and goals, instead of what other people are thinking about you, you would take a giant step toward being that kind of a person.

Relaxing and visualizing are quite natural. There is nothing strange about it. We do it all the time. When we daydream we are relaxing and visualizing. But what kind of daydreams do we have?

How can I get back at him (or her)?

What right has he (or she) to say that to me?

What if I fail?

How am I going to get by on this limited money?

I wonder who he (or she) is with right now?

Please record a few of your daydreams. Relax. Reflect. Write.

These daydreams become learned, too. They are destructive. They teach us fear, worry, insecurity, suspicion, and doubt. These are fattening daydreams. We need to disconnect and to discard these negative, unwanted thoughts forever. We need to connect and to learn different, positive thoughts. We need to develop different, slenderizing daydreams.

Three Ways to Relax for Easy Learning Readiness

When you relax and see (visualize) things happen the way they should happen, you are creating what you want, not what you don't want.

See yourself tormented and you reinforce the torment. See yourself happy and you increase the happiness. *Happiness is a state of mind.* It is a state that only *YOU* can develop and maintain day by day.

The choice is yours. You have chosen to be the way you are even though it seems you have been unlucky or a victim of circumstances.

Well, I have good news for you. You can live life the way you want—as a sufferer or as an enjoyer. All you need to do is to learn how to follow the Schiff plan.

Learning how does not take a college education. It takes a few minutes of relaxing, then picturing or daydreaming (thinking) in a way you have not permitted yourself to do before—in an active, positive, and creative way. Then repetition on a daily basis will bring this picture (these thoughts) into clear focus.

Relax. Picture. Go one day at a time.

Relaxing for most people is not as familiar a procedure as you would think. You know how to relax in front of a television set, and in your head when you go to sleep. But to relax under other, more controlled circumstances, requires assistance.

I'm going to give you three ways to relax. Once you learn how to relax, I will then give you ways to change your eating preferences from wrong to right, and your thoughts from negative to positive.

From then on, it will be clear sailing for you.

1. *Eye Technique.* Sit comfortably in a straight-back chair. Stare at a point on your hand. Don't allow the eyes to blink. When, in a few moments, you feel the need to blink, let your eyes close gently. Let your attention dwell comfortably on your eyes. Be aware of every little sensation in your eye muscles. Coax your eye muscles to relax to the nth degree of perfect comfort. If the eyelids flutter or the eyes water, this is a good sign that your eyes are responding to your instructions. Once delightfully relaxed, send the feeling in them—the liquid comfort—like a wave down your body and all the way to your toes.

2. *Breathing Technique.* Sit comfortably in a straight-back chair. Your legs should be uncrossed, hands on lap. Take a deep breath and, as you exhale, let your eyes close gently. Take a second deep breath and feel your body relaxing from head to toe. Now take a third deep breath. Make it a real deep end-of-the-day sigh and let all your worries and problems be expelled with the air. Sit quietly for a few minutes, allowing your attention to dwell comfortably on your breathing. Feel yourself becoming more and more peaceful and tranquil with every breath you take.

3. *Head-to-Toe Technique.* Sit comfortably as in the previous methods. Let your eyes close gently and permit your attention to drift to your scalp. Check out your scalp for tenseness. Permit the little muscles that control the scalp to relax. When you are sure that your scalp muscles are not taut but are comfortably adjusted, do the same for your forehead. No furrows. No wrinkles. Perfectly smooth. Now your eyes. They may water or your eyelids may flutter. Consider these good signs. How do your face muscles feel? Your mouth? Is your tongue comfortable in your mouth? Perhaps your mouth will water or maybe you will feel the need to swallow. Again, these are good signs. Now move on down to your neck, shoulders, chest. Your arms should feel heavy on your lap. Maybe one feels heavier than the other. Or

perhaps you don't know exactly where your arms are. All good signs. Now relax your stomach, hips, back, thighs, legs, feet, toes. You are now thoroughly relaxed from head to toe.

These are accepted methods for relaxation. They are used in a number of disciplines requiring a state of relaxation, such as meditation, hypnosis, or yoga.

You can select one of these methods, two, or all three. The best thing to do is to use each. At first do each one separately. Do the Eye Technique. A few hours later, do the Breathing Technique. And, maybe the next day, do the Head-to-Toe Technique.

Every time you use one of these techniques, end by saying, "When I open my eyes at the count of three, I will be wide awake and feel better than before." Then count, "One, two, THREE!" If you don't follow this procedure, you could walk about the remainder of the day, yawning and wondering why you are tired. This will be your "coming out" procedure, no matter which method or methods of relaxation you select.

After you have used all three, select the one that is most pleasant and effective for you, the one that feels most natural, consequently more relaxing. Maybe all three feel great. Or maybe one technique does not seem right for you, but the other two are fine. Then eliminate the undesirable method and use the other two. You can use all three if you wish.

If you do so, combine in the order presented: 1, 2 or 1, 3 or 2, 3 and if all three, 1, 2, 3.

How to Give Mental Instructions That Change Eating Habits

If you are relaxed in front of the television set and the commercial comes on, it gives your mind fattening messages and instructions which you obey.

"Buy Mellow Rich Ice Cream—20 delicious flavors."

Perhaps a beautiful female or an attractive male add to the eye appeal. Maybe a family is oohing and aahing over the creamy stuff. But even without these added attractions, you are receiving powerful mental instructions and suggestions to buy that fattening product. And the same goes for Tasty Bread, and Mother Jones' pies—ad infinitum.

Seldom, if ever, do you see a commercial about lamb chops, or chicken, or halibut. So you are being given instructions to eat fast, fattening foods.

These mental instructions work. If you don't believe me, take a look at yourself. The reason they work is that you are relaxed. Without relaxation it requires considerable repetition to get the fattening message across. Through relaxation, plus using your imagination, just a few repeats and the fat cells expand. Unconsciously, with hardly a second thought, you reach for the Mellow Rich Ice Cream, Tasty Bread, and Mother Jones's pies.

Now you are about to use this easy formula (pages 160–2) for your benefit and success instead of being used. You are about to give yourself slenderizing mental instructions while relaxed, thus you will not even see the ice cream, bread, or pie. You will only have eyes for the delicious meats, poultry, fish, and other proteins on the One-Day-At-A-Time Plan plus, of course, the fresh vegetables, greens, salads, and fruits. You will be able to give yourself mental instructions that will make you automatically pass up macaroni and reach instead for the eggs, pass up the crackers and reach instead for the cheese, pass up the potatoes and reach instead for the soy beans, fat-free milk, and other low-fat, low-carbohydrate foods. And the fat cells contract.

These mental instructions are similar to the commercials you see on television. Only you are the announcer. When you are relaxed, you tell yourself what the sponsor wants you to hear.

Only, you are the sponsor. You instruct yourself about your new eating program and how it is totally effective and satisfying.

Here is the basic procedure:

1. You relax using one or more of the techniques provided above.
2. You give yourself mental instructions.
3. You end with the count of three, reminding yourself, "Wide awake! Feeling great!"

You know step 1 and step 3, because you have already practiced them.

Let us talk about step 2. How do you give yourself mental instructions that will make the switching of foods easy, pleasurable, satisfying, and slenderizing?

Actually, it is just like talking to another person. You say what you want to say, clearly and concisely. It is best not to say too much at one time or you will confuse the "other person." The "other person" is, of course, your subconscious mind where all learning resides. You are changing that learning much the same way a computer is given new programming or instructions.

So, as you talk to yourself silently you are slowly changing what your mind has learned and programmed. You must learn to change your mind in order to change your eating habits and control your weight permanently.

Your mind has learned to like sugar and sweets. To change your mind's instructions and learning about sugar is to change your mind about sugar. To change your mind about sugar is to eliminate the craving for sugar.

You say mentally to yourself, while relaxed, "Sugar and sweets bore me. I get more enjoyment from protein foods. Protein foods are good for my body. Foods that are good for my body taste good to me."

Now, there is no right way or wrong to say this to yourself. The words quoted in the above paragraph do not have to be memorized. It is the idea that is important, not the words. Any way that you convey the idea to yourself is fine. Use your own words. Keep them simple. Keep them practical.

You may prefer merely to say, "At every meal I enjoy sweets less and less, protein foods more and more."

Or, "I have less and less desire for sweets, and more and more desire for proteins."

Or, "I want and enjoy whatever is good for me. Sweets are fattening and not healthful for me; proteins are slenderizing and beneficial for me."

The results will be excellent *if* you continue to give yourself positive, clear, mental instructions. Repetition is essential for learning. Repeat again and again.

For instance, "I hate sugar" would *not* be an advisable instruction. "Hate" is a negative, undesirable emotion which saps health and warps the mind. Emphasize the benefits and desire for protein rather than the adverse effects of sugar.

Give yourself positive, clear mental instructions.

Tips for Creating Eating Changes Mentally

A few additional tips for successfully "teaching" your mind new slenderizing ways:

Keep the words literal.
Use mental pictures, too. Visualize. Imagine. Daydream.
Give just a few brief mental instructions each session.
Go one step at a time; one pound at a time; an ounce at a time.

So we use positive concepts. We use common words that are not ambiguous and spell out exactly what we intend to create. We do not attempt to remember or to say too much at each relaxation session. And we don't strive to go all the way in one session. Haste makes waste.

Literal words are necessary because the subconscious mind takes everything literally. You would not say, for instance, "I will like proteins, dislike sugar." The word "will" refers to the future. The future never comes. Keep the instructions in the present. "I like protein. I dislike sugar." Or, "I like to feel comfortable. I dislike feeling stuffed." And so on.

Let me skip to the fourth tip, "Go one step at a time." If you like sugar and say "I dislike sugar," the little old computer we call the subconscious mind will usually reject this instruction:

"DOES NOT COMPUTE." "IS NONSENSIBLE." "DOES NOT WORK." "REJECTED."

So you need to go one small step at a time: "I like sugar less and less. I like protein foods more and more. I like overeating and fatty foods less and less. I love me more and more."

"DOES COMPUTE." "IS SENSIBLE." "DOES WORK." "ACCEPTED."

I have already discussed not attempting to remember too much at a single session. Brief mental instructions are good because they are easier to recall. Anything requiring excessive mental exertion interferes with deep relaxation.

So let us look at that remaining tip, "Use mental pictures, too." If you picture yourself not attached to sugar and sweets but enjoying fish, chicken, and meat instead, you are reinforcing verbal statements a hundredfold!

And that's conservative. The Chinese say that a picture is worth a thousand words. Maybe so. Certainly mental pictures are powerful mental instructions, especially when repeated day after day.

Always include a mental picture of yourself eating the way you are instructing yourself to eat. Or behaving emotionally in the way you will be instructing yourself to be, which we will cover in this chapter.

Now, here are some additional verbal instructions that will help ensure your quick and easy success on the One-Day-At-A-Time program.

Words—"I need the empty calories in sweets and starchy foods less and less. I enjoy nutritional foods, high in protein, high in minerals, and high in vitamins—more and more."

Picture—See yourself passing up cola or cookies and "lighting up" as you enjoy meats, fish, chicken, salads. See yourself slim.

Words—"I need fatty food less and less. I enjoy skim milk, skinless chicken, low-fat cheeses, and lean meat more and more."

Picture—See yourself drinking skim milk, relishing cottage cheese, cutting the skin off chicken and the fat off meat. See yourself free of fat.

Words—"Higher nutrition in the protein foods on my slenderizing program are so satisfactory that I derive adequate enjoyment with smaller portions."

Picture—See yourself eating your favorite meat, fish, or poultry and being satisfied with a modest portion. See yourself thin and attractive.

Words—"Because I eat two more meals on my slenderizing program, I have little need to eat between meals."

Picture—See yourself going through the day with the clock showing the time at each meal and no other eating taking place. See yourself slimmer.

Words—"My body needs liquid. I drink eight glasses of liquid a day, mostly water. Whenever I feel the urge to eat in between meals, a glass of cold water satisfies that desire."

Picture—See yourself drinking eight times a day with a calendar showing today's date. Include coffee, tea, low-calorie soda, unsweetened juice, but lots of water. See yourself walking by the refrigerator to drink water at the sink instead. See yourself as slender and attractive.

Words—"I relax every day and give myself positive, clear instructions for correct eating and thinking. Each time I do, I relax more deeply, self-instruct more effectively, and feel better and better."

Picture—See yourself in your usual chair, relaxing. See yourself radiant, beaming, healthy, slender.

Tips for Creating Higher Levels of Well-Being Mentally

These words and pictures are powerful tools when you use them while relaxed. The more you use them the easier and more natural it will be for you to eat in a slenderizing and enjoyable way.

Remember, *ease* and *enjoyment* are the key to success on the One-Day-At-A-Time Plan.

Another key is the recognition and understanding of emotional reasons for wanting to eat when not hungry, for wanting to feed your appetite (your false hunger).

Your writing will be like a window to your soul. The recognition and understanding are already taking place if you have begun to write.

Now you need to help yourself to switch thoughts, emotions, and attitudes.

Just the way words and mental pictures help you to switch away from those two white foods, sugar and flour, words and mental pictures can help you to switch away from those dark thoughts and turbulent emotions.

Willpower *is not* enough.

Emil Coué, the French author who made the affirmation popular, "Every day in every way I am getting better and better," also said, "When the will and the imagination are in conflict, it is always the imagination that wins."

"I will lose weight." You can fix this thought and desire in your mind with the help of your imagination day by day. Repetition is important. You will succeed sooner than you thought possible.

You can resolve not to eat any more, but if you picture that leftover pie in the refrigerator, your resolve is as good as gone. You resist. You resist another few minutes. Eventually the mental picture wins and you help yourself to the pictured pie.

Now you need to help yourself to a different mental picture, different in many ways.

In addition to pie not being in this new picture, negative, unwanted thoughts, emotions, and attitudes are also not in the picture.

All too often we have "put down" thoughts about ourselves. We feel inadequate. We feel limited. We feel unattractive. We feel poor. We feel insecure. We feel let down. And we put ourselves down. The only "up thing" is our weight.

And we eat. The food temporarily blocks these thoughts, feelings, and attitudes of inadequacy. We substitute food for love and lack of self-love.

This self-concept or self-image is there constantly. It is instructing our mind to behave in the way we see and believe ourselves to be.

Usually this image agrees with past instructions we have received from a source we respect and believe. So, as a child, when our mother or father, our loved ones or peers called us "Stupid!" and "Clumsy!", we accepted these characteristics as true. They became part of our self-image. We made them part of our self-image. And we lived that way.

And we lived to eat.

We continue to take things personally and embellish this self-portrait. "I can't do this, I'm a failure at that."

A self-portrait that shows us wanting and lacking programs (instructs) us to live as the person that we see and believe ourselves to be. A self-portrait of a person short on attributes is a fattening self-portrait.

As we see and believe ourselves to be a small person in capability, we seem to compensate by being a big person in body. Subtract from the ego, add to the body. And the only thing that adds up is your weight.

We need to change our self-image—beautify it, upgrade it—improve it day by day.

Stacy R., 32, was a backslider. She would go on the One-Day Plan and, finding herself enjoying it immensely, she would continue to eat that way. Then something would happen in her life and back she would slide on slippery sweets and starches.

For instance, a well-meaning friend, who offered her chocolate and was refused, reminded her how her sister had died while dieting, taking nonprescription diet pills in excessive amounts. Immediately, she felt guilty at not having succeeded in helping her sister. She gave in to the emotional blackmail and ate the chocolate.

There were many similar experiences that caused backsliding. She would lose weight, then gain it back. This happened for the first month or so on the program. She did not change much from her original 151 pounds.

Then she began to understand from her writing exactly what was happening. She revealed a pattern of triggering events that caused self-pity, or guilt, or some other self-image destroyer.

Once recognized and understood, she was able to give herself the kind of positive instructions that immunized her from disruptive events and emotional blackmail.

Four months later at 115 pounds, she wrote, "I have had miraculous results. I think about and understand myself. I am more aware of what is happening. The most important thing—I have learned to really like myself. That sounds simple to do. But it is not. I have a couple of pounds to lose to reach my desired weight. I know I will get there. And I know I will stay there for the rest of my life."

Words and Pictures That Create a Slender Self-Image

You *need* to begin with positive, clear, concise, self-image words and mental pictures. You *need* to relax and instruct yourself with words and mental pictures that you are a capable, lovable, creative, important person. The most important person in your lifetime—YOU.

Then you can go on to give yourself specific mental instructions that end the dark thoughts, negative attitudes, and distressed emotions which you have identified in your writing. Replace them with light thoughts, positive attitudes, and uplifting emotions.

Again, the procedure is:

1. Relax, using any one or more techniques as before (pages 160–2).

2. Give yourself words and see pictures that move you to positive, high-spirited living (pages 166–7).

3. End your session at the count of three, feeling great.

It is not magic, but it works like magic. The words are not mystic incantations, but the way they whisk away mental clouds, they could very well be a kind of abracadabra.

It is all so simple that it makes you wonder why people tolerate fears and phobias, morose and depressed moods, worry and anxiety. It is as if this is their choice, a dull and dreary choice. Certainly it is not an intelligent choice, and it is often a fatty choice.

As a physician and bariatrician, I know how important this emotional switch is. I see disease after disease caused by stress. It appears that the difference between a sick person and a well person is *how* that person reacts to life's problems; to their problems; to themselves.

Worry equals sickness, dis-ease, lack of mental (emotional) and spiritual ease. Confidence and self-assurance equals health, ease, mental (emotional) equilibrium, and spiritual enlightenment.

Can you decide which equals overweight and which equals slender?

Begin now to enjoy relaxation sessions to start a love affair with yourself. Here are the kinds of words and mental pictures you can use to trigger the romance.

Words—"I can do whatever I decide to do. I am capable and effective."

Picture—See yourself with your goal accomplished.

Words—"I am honest and sincere, intelligent and efficient."

Picture—See yourself being awarded a plaque with that inscription on it.

Words—"I have more and more confidence in myself with every passing day and know that I have talents not yet fully used."

Picture—See yourself walking tall and proud.

Who do you understand yourself to be? How much do you like (love) yourself? What are your good points? Are you thinking thin?

Open your book "ME" and answer the above questions. Write your own words, words that upgrade your self-concept. These will be words on a page, but they will help create your slender, alluring self.

Words and Pictures That Brighten Dismal Thoughts

As you are now is a result of your old self-portrait. As you will now become will be a result of your new self-portrait.

Here are six unwanted, fattening factors in the old self-portrait and their desirable slenderizing substitutes in the new self-portrait:

Old Self-Portrait	New Self-Portrait
1. Overweight	1. Slim
2. Eats sweets, starches and fat	2. Enjoys proteins and nutritious foods

3. Problem-prone
4. Dislikes self
5. Sluggish and unattractive
6. Negative in thoughts, attitudes, and feelings

3. Success-prone
4. Loves and admires self
5. Energetic and attractive
6. Positive in thoughts, attitudes, and feelings

I have given you the words and pictures for factors 1, 2, 3, 4, and 5. Now we need to examine the kinds of words and pictures that create a new self-portrait for factor 6—thoughts, attitudes, and feelings.

There are general, positive words and pictures that improve the emotional climate, such as Emile Coué's "Every day in every way I'm getting better and better." These are words that zero in on nervousness, frustration, anxiety, loneliness, and worry. They move you instead into tranquility, understanding, confidence, self-sufficiency, optimism—and weight loss.

"I am tranquil. I am understanding." These are good, positive words. They help everyone, no matter what their specific problems may include. These are slenderizing words. But by zeroing in on a specific problem as you write to yourself or to me, you use words and pictures that are meaningful to you, and to your unwanted pounds.

I can give you words and mental pictures for general instructions. We will use the five general emotional conditions mentioned above with their "word and picture" counterpart detailed below. However, I cannot possibly list all the specific instructions targeted for every problem that besets the overweight person. These problems come in all shapes, sizes, and forms as different as the overweight persons themselves.

But I will give you a few examples later. You will see by the five general instructions, and the later examples of specific instructions, what you need to do to put together words and mental pictures to use in your ending of specific problem emotions and negative attitudes.

First the general instructions:

NERVOUSNESS, RESTLESSNESS

Words—"I am growing stronger every day and more and more in control. I am becoming more serene, tranquil, and calm. I am patient and composed."

Picture—See yourself unmoved by agitation; holding the tiller of your ship steady despite rough seas. See yourself as a pillar of strength.

FRUSTRATION, ANGER

Words—"I am insulated from the irrational behavior of others. It is their problem, not mine, and I am not the target. I am calm, cool, collected, and in control of my emotions."

Picture—See yourself with a plastic bubble around you. Barbs hit it and bounce away. See yourself smiling and understanding in all situations.

UPSET, ANXIOUS

Words—"Things are not as bad as they often look. I see the good side. I remain positive and confident in the face of what appears to be adversity."

Picture—See yourself brimming with confidence at the outset of upsetting circumstances. See the circumstances change. See your confidence rewarded by the outcome.

LONELY, INSECURE

Words—"I am self-sufficient and capable. I am desirable as a person and confident that I am attracting who is right for me. I am secure in my philosophy and religious beliefs."

Picture—See yourself as an ideal companion. See all your needs being met.

WORRY, FEAR

Words—"There is nothing to fear. I divest myself of all fear and worry. I am more and more optimistic and joyful. I'm confident I'll achieve my final weight, one day at a time."

Picture—See yourself in a fearless posture. See yourself radiating confidence and joy to your family, co-workers, and friends. See yourself slender and attractive.

Remember, it does no good to read this. You *must* set the book aside, then relax and say these words, holding in your mind these pictures. Repetition will focus, develop, and fix the picture onto your mental screen.

The positive results catapult your spirits up and your weight down.

Specific Instructions for Special Conditions

"I have built walls of fat around myself—for self-defense," writes Gail W. "I have such a great fear of my alcoholic ex-husband being attracted to me."

Gail, in her late thirties, weighed 223 pounds when I first saw her. Nearly three years later, she was back weighing 32 pounds less. Not much progress. But one reason was, she had not made much progress with her emotional problems. Spinning wheels. Playing games.

Her mother was a brain damaged deaf-mute. Gail became an alcoholic in her teens. She went through two marriages with alcoholic men, both prolonged traumatic experiences.

While she lost 32 pounds, albeit over three years, she eliminated the drinking habit. I considered that worth all the weight loss she had not attained. Now, at least, she had a longer life ahead in which to enjoy her approaching slenderness.

I convinced Gail to write more and to give herself specific instructions.

She wrote, "I will overcome these fears about my ex-husband, men and myself. I believe in the spiritual power of God . . . I will develop patience . . . And I will attain my weight goal by next June in time for my son's graduation."

I did not have to give Gail the specific instructions to use during her relaxed periods. She derived them from her own writing:

Words—"I am working out my fears. I am patient. I place my faith in God and in myself."

Picture—She saw herself fearless and staunch in her resolve. She saw the calendar marked June and the scale at 150.

Gail attended her son's graduation a more slender person—weight 156 pounds and still descending.

As you write, you gain enlightenment. Enlightenment gained is tantamount to weight loss. One specific reason is that it gives you the words and pictures you need to instruct your mind to switch from negative to positive polarity, from weight-gaining feelings and negative behavior to weight-loss feelings and positive behavior.

Suppose you were afraid of losing the sale whenever you dealt with a customer. So you ate before and after each instance. You did not connect the doughnuts, pie, cake, candy, beer, and whiskey sours with this lack of sales confidence, but now you have written about your inner feelings and this has all come to light. What do you do about it?

You need to give your mind new instructions about your sales ability:

Words—"I am knowledgeable about the products (or services) I sell. I can communicate their benefits to a potential customer. This means I am a successful salesperson. I am convincing and capable."

Picture—You see yourself making sale after sale. Customers are happy and returning. New customers arrive. Happy days.

Suppose you have aches and pains. Some of them are suspiciously close to your heart area. However, your physician gives you a clean bill of health, except a reminder that you should lose 20 to 30 pounds, and be better off for it.

But the aches and pains persist. Could your physician be wrong? Do you have some deadly disease? Better live it up. You eat and drink all the food and drink you don't need.

What words do you use and what pictures do you hold in your mind as you relax and change this behavior through positive mental instructions?

Consider using these:

Words—"My health is getting better and better. I sleep well, breathe fresh air, and eat proteins and other nutritious food. My body grows stronger and stronger."

Picture—You see yourself radiant with health, free of pain, vibrant with energy. You see yourself eating for health and nutrition, becoming more youthful and physically more powerful.

It is simple to relax and give yourself the proper mental instructions.

It is so simple and the changes that occur are so dramatic that you cannot afford to let another minute go by. It is this moment, this hour, this One Day that really counts.

X

ACCELERATING A NEW ATTRACTIVE LOOK

Your physical body is what I am interested in as a physician, but the mental "body" controls and shapes your physical body. So, I must not ignore your mental well-being if I am to be of physical help to you. The body dances to whatever tune the mind plays. Learn to play beautiful music.

In the previous chapter we learned how to give ourselves mental instructions to change our mental "body." We called that mental body our self-image or self-concept and we worked on it as if it were a self-portrait.

We learned how to relax and give ourselves mental instructions to change all aspects of that self-portrait. (Pages 171-172.)

We still have additional, important work to do on No. 5 of the self-portrait or self-image, our ego structure or "inner being."

You must change from the usual sluggish and unattractive physical traits of an overweight person to the vigorous, straight posture and attractive exuberance of a slender person.

In this chapter, you will learn secrets that will help you accelerate your transformation from fat to thin.

You will learn how to move, stand, think, walk, act, and do in ways that help the body to become what you want it to be—its natural, slender silhouette. The first step will be to prepare your mind for the changes that are about to occur.

You are going to change your mind about your body.

To change your mind about your body is to change your body.

To change your mind and body permanently is to eliminate the unwanted pounds forever!

You are going to instruct your mind to alter your dimensions and physical contour.

Enter your present measurements in the book, "ME."

Now enter your desired measurements. Please don't be vague.

Be sure to include neck, arms, bust or chest, abdomen, waist, hips, thighs, calves.

Now do the following exercise:

1. Relax, using the procedures practiced in the last chapter, but holding your book in your lap, open to your dimensions.

2. Open your eyes and read your present measurements. Close your eyes and say, "I reject them." See yourself as you are and put a big red "X" over the picture. REJECTED! DOES NOT COMPUTE.

3. Open your eyes again and read your desired measurements. Close your eyes and say, "I come closer to these smaller measurements with every passing day." See yourself as you desire to be. Know that you can fulfill this desire eventually—you will not fail yourself. ACCEPTED! DOES COMPUTE.

Some Changes That Are About to Occur

Please reflect upon subtle or obvious changes that are occurring within you. If you experience too much difficulty, you are reminded how important it is to review this book and to follow its instructions.

We learn by relaxing, using the imagination, reinforced by repetition day by day. As you spend these quiet moments with yourself—and just two or three times a day is sufficient—relaxing, imagining, and repeatedly giving your mind these instructions, you begin to change.

Let me give you just one example of something that has already begun to take place, having progressed this far in the book—you no longer have the carefree attitude you had a few days ago about sugar and sweet products. You are also beginning to look at bread, cake, and other white flour products more as an enemy than a friend. Choose your friends carefully.

These are valuable changes. They are worth much more to you in pounds lost than ten days or more of a starvation diet.

Because I have insisted you read this book before beginning the Schiff Plan, you have experienced a switch in attitude toward sweets, starches, and fat that will be reinforced on the One-Day-At-A-Time program and perpetuated long after.

Just reading this book is triggering these changes. But I have insisted on three additional, important activities:

1. Preparing a notebook called "ME."
2. Writing in your notebook about your activities and yourself day by day.
3. Relaxing, imagining, and giving your mind instructions via a plan or program (this book).

If, besides reading this book, you are performing these three additional activities, the changes that are now unfolding in you are quite likely the most significant that could happen in your life. Continue, and you'll make them happen gradually—one day at a time.

As you see yourself thinner, your mind begins to make you thinner. Your mind is the center of your universe and its power is infinite and unlimited—you alone can diminish or increase it.

You move like a thin person.
You talk like a thin person.
You act and do like a thin person.
Look for these changes in yourself. You will see them happening.

What do I mean "move" like a thin person?

A thin person is more mobile than an overweight person. Even if you carry only 20 or 30 pounds excess baggage, you cannot move as freely in comparison to the lesser weight.

A person who is overweight is really older than a person of the identical age who is slender. Excess pounds decrease your life expectancy. You feel older than a slender person of the same age.

Give yourself mental instructions that make you more of a mobile youthful person. Choose one or more of these or compose you own:

Words—"I feel more youthful. I have more spring in my step."

Picture—See yourself walking briskly, bounding up the steps, moving at a less burdened clip.

Words—"Movement helps my circulation and so nourishes my body. I help my body to feed all tissues and organs by this rejuvenating motion."

Picture—See yourself walking instead of riding, participating in more activities, going on picnics, spending an afternoon at the beach, or doing whatever you enjoy. See yourself looking younger.

Words—"Exercise burns fat. As I exercise more and more I become more slender."

Picture—See yourself bowling, riding a bicycle, jogging a few steps, swimming, playing ping pong, or any other sport or games you enjoy. See your measurements decreasing. See your physical being decreasing.

Enjoyment is the key. Do not instruct your mind to go on picnics if you can't stand ants or insects. Instruct your mind in positive, enthusiastic, and enjoyable ways that add to your fun in life.

It is fun to be an active, thin person. Start being active, as though you were thin again. Think thin. Act thin. Be thin.

How To Burn Off Pounds Without Exerting Yourself

I am not an outspoken proponent of jogging a few miles a day nor do I prescribe vigorous calisthenics. Jogging is fine, if you enjoy jogging. Push-ups and jumping jacks are fine, if you enjoy them.

What you enjoy and therefore do regularly is ten times more effective for you than something you do not enjoy and unwillingly have to discipline yourself to do. Unplanned and ineffective discipline fails. Enjoyment succeeds.

You can help those disappearing pounds to depart faster by enjoyable movements. And playing your favorite game of cricket several times a day will cause more pounds to melt away in your lifetime than forcing yourself to jog, knowing it is not your "thing." Eventually the forced activity will stop and the pounds reappear.

Moving feels good and is good for you. It feels good to stretch. It feels good to get out of a chair you have been sitting in for a long time. It feels good to walk off a meal, perspire a bit, play an active game, exercise. The good feeling that movement brings means that your body relishes it. Movement aids the circulation, tones the muscles, and improves the complexion.

Stretching does not have to be confined to your bed on arising in the morning. You can stretch your legs sitting; you can stretch your arms at your desk; you can arch your back waiting for the bus, you can stretch your neck and torso while driving.

If you are aware of the good feeling this stretching brings, I don't have to tell you when and where to do it. You will become a persistent, innovative, ubiquitous stretcher.

If you are aware of the good feeling that a walk produces, you will be taking more strolls, brisk walks, and perhaps walking somewhere instead of driving.

If you are aware of the good feeling that comes with flexing a muscle, you will put one hand or arm against the other in different positions whenever you have a moment. You will also move your body in various ways when alone to flex muscles that are crying "me too."

My program succeeds because it is a total, comprehensive program geared to *you*—your food likes and dislikes, your thinking, your life-style problems, your self-image, and your body. It is a "Holistic Program." It is mind-body oriented. It is YOU oriented.

From food to motion, the emphasis is on you. If I pick the food for you, color it failure. If I pick the motion for you, color it failure also.

You pick the food. You enjoy the food. Color it success. You pick the physical movements. You enjoy the motion. Color it pounds-off success. Learn to pick—and enjoy yourself.

How to Renew Weight Loss Once You Hit a Plateau

Changes have already begun. As you read this book and write in your book called "ME," you change. But changes officially commence on that One Day. And they continue thereafter.

I have said before that you may wish to repeat the One-Day-At-A-Time Plan, or you may continue without knowingly making a decision. It may instinctively become your life style. Either way, the changes in your weight continue. The changes in your measurements continue. The changes in your level of happiness continue. The changes in your movements and activities continue. The changes in you continue day after day.

But sometimes the changes taper off. This is natural. What is also natural—but a natural error—is for you to become discouraged when this happens.

Discouragement is fattening. It can potentially contain more calories than a carload of you know what.

Do not allow yourself to become discouraged when your weight reaches a plateau—when the weight loss slows down, stops, and does not start again. Discouragement is a "cop-out"! Plateaus are natural periods of metabolic, chemical, energy (food-intake, exercise), and emotional adjustments.

Never become discouraged. Instead, continue *and* increase the work on your self-image, on your writing, on the perfection of your recipes and menus, on the many aspects of your plan. Eventually the plateau will end and your weight loss will resume.

Robin J., middle-aged real estate agent, went on the Schiff Plan and found herself approaching her weight goal in just a few months.

Then the weight loss stopped and she became discouraged, too discouraged to come back to the office for further advice. She had regained most of the excess weight before she finally returned.

I had her begin my plan again, only this time I prepared her for the weight-loss plateau that she could experience again. I'll let Robin tell you the rest of her story:

"In the past, whenever I hit a 'Plateau' and the needle on my scale would not move, I would grow discouraged. And the easiest thing in the world to do was to console myself with some 'forbidden fruit.' Now I can look at the scale and know that I have followed the program and have done the required thinking and writing. If I stay on the program and continue my 'activities' day by day, the needle on the scale will move eventually. I'm still making mistakes, but I'm learning to recognize and correct them. I plan to reach my goal, and this time I'll continue at my goal weight."

Robin did just that and all it necessitated was not allowing herself to become discouraged.

If the needle on your scale takes a rest during its trip down, do not love yourself less. Love yourself more. Write, think, and learn more about yourself. Do more for yourself—use and apply the instructions in this book, daily.

Relax, imagine, and give yourself positive, uplifting mental instructions.

Know that the needle will start moving again *only* when you start moving again—mentally, emotionally, spiritually.

Another common mistake: trying harder.

Do not try harder.

Trying is working against yourself. The effort is futile. Spinning wheels. Playing games—the "Merry-Go-Round," the "Yo-Yo" game. Failing—sooner or later. Work for yourself. Rev-up your optimism and enthusiasm. Learn to cooperate with yourself. Do this while enjoying life more in the program by using and applying on a daily basis the information and instructions in this book.

Accelerating a New Attractive Look 181

Robin was eating the same foods day in and day out. I had her make up a week of menus to make each day more enjoyable.

You will find Robin's week on pages 182 and 183.

By breaking out of the humdrum of eating the same food each day, Robin also broke out of the humdrum of frequent plateaus. Eating became more fun. She even allowed more time from her busy real estate day to prepare interesting menus.

What is humdrum for you may be exciting for someone else and vice versa. You need to "do your thing," measuring it by your own "kiks."

A plateau is a "rut." To break out of any "rut" you must change direction.

To change the direction of your physical weight and to eliminate those unwanted pounds permanently, you must change foods, food preparation, portion size, eating behavior, and food-related patterns.

The Magic Formula for Continuing Weight Loss

Recently 100 obesity experts convened in Bethesda, Maryland for a conference on weight control sponsored by the National Institute of Health.

They discussed the growing problem. They agreed on a number of facts about overweight people:

About 25% of the population is overweight.

More money is spent on worthless "cures" than all medical research combined.

Overweight is associated with diabetes, heart disease, high blood pressure, gall bladder disease, cancer of the uterus, plus many other medical conditions.

The level of fatness in women decreases as education and income rise.

Men lose more years off their life because of excess pounds than do women.

Black women tend to be more overweight than white women, but black men are leaner than white men.

But what the conference could not agree on was any specific way to handle the overweight problem. Perhaps the one concept which seemed to be most uniformly accepted was:

	BREAKFAST	LUNCH	DINNER	SNACKS
MONDAY	6 ozs. unsweetened grapefruit juice 1 boiled egg 1 slice melba toast Black coffee with artificial sweetener	Green salad with diet dressing Diet cola ½ small apple	4 oz. pattie ground beef Zucchini (steamed) 1 glass of non-fat milk	½ apple
TUESDAY	½ cantaloupe filled with low-fat cottage cheese Black coffee	Tuna salad Sliced tomatoes Diet cola	Squash casserole**	Celery Sticks Pickles
WEDNESDAY	Orange juice—fresh squeezed with liquid protein Black coffee	Liquid protein Diet cola	Baked chicken breast Broccoli Non-fat milk D-Zerta jello Black coffee	Cheese—low fat
THURSDAY	Scrambled eggs with mushrooms Tomato juice Black coffee	Non-fat milk Carrot sticks Apple (small) (ate at desk)	6 oz. steak—broiled Steamed spinach	(Went bowling—no snack)

Accelerating a New Attractive Look

FRIDAY	Grapefruit juice—natural packed with liquid protein Black coffee	Chef salad Bleu cheese dressing (ate with client) Black coffee	Small broiled lamb chop Broiled mushrooms Steamed chard Black coffee	Cantaloupe
SATURDAY	Grapefruit juice with liquid protein Black coffee	Spinach salad with hard-boiled egg and sliced mushrooms	Squash Casserole** Black coffee	Carrots Celery Radishes
SUNDAY	Orange juice Omelet with cottage cheese Black coffee	Tossed green salad with diet dressing Diet cola	Roast leg of lamb Yellow squash String beans Non-fat milk Coffee	Cheese Casaba melon

**Squash Casserole

1 medium onion	2 eggs, well beaten
1 T oil	½ C grated cheese
2 C cooked mashed squash	Salt substitute and pepper

(Robin used summer squash. It is less starchy than Hubbard or winter squash.)

Brown onion in oil until tender. Pour into bowl with squash. Stir in eggs and seasoning and ⅔ of the cheese. Pour into casserole. Sprinkle remaining cheese over top. Bake at 350 degrees for one hour. Serves 4–6.

Weight loss without rehabilitation of life style is fruitless because you gain it all back—sooner or later.

The *only way* not to gain it back is to change your life style, day by day. What is life style? Eating, thinking, understanding, self-instructing, enjoying, learning, doing, and being.

Eat, think, understand and instruct differently; then enjoying, learning, doing, and being automatically follow in their wake.

You must learn to change your life style day by day in order to change your eating habits and control your weight—permanently!

I am not asking you to resolve to lose weight. I am not asking you to set an unrealistic and self-defeating goal to lose a certain amount of pounds by a certain date. I am not asking you to use unplanned, ineffective discipline and illogical, self-deceiving willpower. I am not asking you to make useless and meaningless sacrifices in your eating enjoyment. I am not asking you to count calories or amounts of food. I am not asking you to starve yourself or to diet per se.

All I am asking you to do is to switch certain foods and switch certain thoughts, one day at a time.

Then you will have changed your life style.

You will live as a new person—becoming slender and remaining that way—always.

How to Keep Problems from Triggering Appetite

One of my patients had a traumatic experience. She was beaten and raped. It caused her to go into seclusion. Her weight increased. When she came to me she did lots of writing about that experience and problem. She began to handle the terrible memory of the event. She could begin to relate to other people. She returned to work.

Then she had problems with her supervisor. She began to "drown" these problems with food and drink—the wrong kind of food and the wrong kind of drink. When she returned for help, twenty lost pounds had been regained.

"What do I do now?" was her plaintive appeal.

Some problems are so evident that they do not need identification—just patience, thought, and understanding. Writing alone will not lead to the disconnection between problems and food. What will accomplish that disconnection is the understanding about other people and their problems. When they react negatively to you, they are often complaining about their own problems, not about you.

This patient's supervisor was not intentionally hassling her, but merely expressing a hidden personal problem. The patient, taking it personally, was creating a nonexistent problem and taking to food as consolation.

I explained the problem to her. She seemed to understand. I advised her to become involved in different activities and ways to release pent-up, frustrated feelings instead of eating and overeating whenever these hassles occurred.

She wrote, but she also did other things, such as reorganizing her kitchen and revarnishing the cabinets. Whenever she returned home after an annoying day, she headed straight for the kitchen as usual, but instead of eating she worked.

It was good therapy. She lost those twenty pounds again. Meanwhile, her supervisor was transferred to another division.

We all carry our problems with us wherever we go. Problems at home are carried to work. Problems at work are carried home.

Disconnect problems from food. Don't reach for food. Learn to resolve your problems through common sense and understanding. You can give your mind instructions to lay these problems aside, knowing they will be there waiting for you whenever you decide to think about them.

Stress causes more than overweight itself. It saps resistance and strains vital organs. You can cut stress in half by separating work from home life. Here are the instructions to give yourself while blissfully relaxed.

Words—"When I leave work, I leave work problems. They no longer are part of my life. I have other important things to do."

Picture—See yourself involved in some project the moment you arrive home, such as weeding the lawn, painting the house, or loving your spouse.

Words—"When I leave home, I leave family problems. They no longer are part of my life. My work effectivness is my priority."

Picture—See yourself doing your job efficiently without any thought of home life. You are a part of an organization or firm. You serve your organization and humanity. Indirectly, but significantly, you also serve yourself as your weight decreases.

How to Change the Subject and Change Yourself

Activity is great medicine. Feeling sorry for yourself or feeling animosity toward someone is poison. Activity is the antidote.

I have already given you gentle ways to be more physically active, but now I am referring to activities which keep you mentally active. When your mind hangs on to a problem, change the subject. And don't accept food as a change of subject. You are chewing over the same problem. And the problem becomes weighty.

Here are a number of examples of different activities:

Phone your stockbroker.
Chit-chat with a friend.
Make love.
Make any kind of joy.
Count to 100.
Count your money.
Count your blessings.
Take a look in a full-length mirror.
Take a shower, or soak in the tub.
Take a swim.
Look out the window.
Daydream.
Stargaze.
Meditate.
Drink water, decaffeinated coffee, or other permitted beverages.
Chew gum (sugarless).
Ride a bike or a horse or take a drive.
Play the piano, a harmonica, etc.
Sing or hum a tune.
Water the lawn.
Trim the flowers.
Enjoy nature.
Go to a library.
Read a book.
Go to a health club, gym, or sauna.
Take a course.
Find a second job.

Visit a friend.
Go to the park or a concert.
Walk the dog.
Walk the kids.
Take a hike.
Paint, sew, crochet, knit, etc.
Do an errand.
Do a good deed.
Do calisthenics.
Walk.
Run.
Go to a movie.
Go dancing.
Write a poem.
Visit your church or temple.
Listen to another person's problems.

In other words, change the subject. Notice I'm not recommending that you go out for a soda or a pizza. Even if food is talked about, change the subject.

Disconnect problems from food. Substitute some other mind-occupying activity in its place. The switch in activity will activate a switch in your weight. And the switch will activate a slimmer you.

Just searching for your sugarless gum, extracting a slice, peeling off the wrapper, and feeling the new taste spring into your mouth with the first movement of your jaw can take your mind off your problem momentarily. Then, perhaps other thoughts will develop and take over. If, on the other hand, the problem pops back, change the subject again. Play gin rummy with a friend.

Food as a Method of Self-Punishment

Jill V., 39, whose field was psychology and sociology, had practiced yoga, meditation, assertive training, and a number of other behavioral techniques.

Yet, when it came to writing and analyzing her own weight problem, she balked. It required a lot of encouragement on my part, but it finally paid off. The following revelations surfaced in Jill as she wrote:

"The first time I wrote, it was almost defiantly. OK, Doctor, I wrote, now let's see what happens. It was truly amazing. I started thinking about what I wrote. Suddenly, I realized it was 9 P.M. and I had not had the urge to eat. I had been busy using my time constructively and I laughed at how fast it went by and how easily my urge to eat had disappeared. What had I written? I wrote about my frustration with the Doctor who did not tell me what and how much to eat, and how to diet. I realized I wanted to punish myself with a diet; to be bored, deprived. So I ate lettuce and cottage cheese, lettuce and cottage cheese. My mind developed 'tunnel vision.' I did not eat anything I enjoyed. I became bored, frustrated, angry. I wanted pills. I wanted the Doctor to do it for me.

"Then I heard your voice explaining that it was my responsibility and I had to do it myself. I remembered you stressing that my problems concern both the physical and the mental weight. Also, the solutions include both food and 'food for thought.' I realized I was not applying my own psychological knowledge to myself. I was torturing myself with food and diet.

"I realized I was the same as the drug addicts I had been helping. A food addict, using it to combat anger, depression, frustration, and other negative feelings and attitudes.

"Me? Depressed? My staunch German upbringing? My professionalism? I realized I was avoiding myself in the thought area, and punishing myself for it in the food area."

Jill jumped into the program full swing from that moment on and used her psychological skills to face up to her guilt feelings and untoward attitudes. End of one more weight problem.

More often we find food being used as a reward rather than a punishment. But the latter is prevalent, too. And we need to be aware of this possibility in ourselves.

Are you feeling guilty about something? Are those second and third portions like tastes of a whip to get even with yourself? Write in "ME" and read the answer.

Feeling guilty about overeating and being overweight can cause additional overeating and overweight. Guilt is fattening.

Handle it by learning to forgive, understand, accept, and like

Accelerating a New Attractive Look

yourself. Relax, imagine, and give yourself new mental instructions.

Words—"I no longer desire to feel guilty. I appreciate myself. I know myself better day by day. The better I know myself, the more I understand and like myself."

Picture—See yourself on trial. See the foreman of the jury handing the verdict to the judge. Hear the judge say "Not guilty." People hug you. You feel cleansed of all guilt. You feel good about yourself.

A reminder that the suggested words and pictures I give you are not required procedures. You can use your own words and your own pictures. In fact, it is desirable that you provide them in accordance with your vocabulary and your own symbols, tailoring them to fit your own situation and life style.

Emergency Measures That Deal Harshly with Fattening Foods and Fattening Thoughts

If, despite improvements in your eating and thinking habits, there are still specific foods that "enslave" you and specific thoughts that "bug" you, you may have to take some harsh means to deal with these culprits.

Suppose, for instance, you have switched from sweets and starches to proteins and greens, but you become like putty every time chocolate cake is within reach. You cannot pass it up. You are on your second slice before the others have finished cutting their first. And in order to appear beneficent, you offer to "share the last piece with someone."

How do you get chocolate cake to "toe the line" along with the other sweets and starches? When you relax deeply, using the techniques I have given you, there is an extremely close relationship between you and your behaving, thinking brain. Your instructions act as commands.

Now, these commands can be based on fact or fantasy. Your mind will still obey, just like a reliable computer. It is similar to a computer. A computer can be programmed with wrong information and it will still work, giving back the exact wrong information you fed into it.

You can give your mind instructions that will change how something tastes, feels, or smells. A person under deep hypnotic relaxation can be told ammonia smells like perfume and he or she will breathe it in deeply and, instead of choking up, will want a second smell.

If you are able to relax deeply, you can tell yourself that chocolate cake tastes like castor oil. Or that cigarette smoke smells like burnt rubber. Or that ice cream turns into fat as it trickles down your throat.

These are called obnoxious techniques. As I mentioned before, we prefer positive instructions. These are negative.

But if all sweets and starches have bowed out in favor of the allowable foods, except chocolate cake for example, it is perhaps the lesser of the two evils to use negative instructions rather than succumb as a cake-a-holic. So, you relax. You imagine you are home in your living room. The doorbell rings. Your neighbor has brought you a chocolate cake she just baked "especially for you." You picture yourself setting it down in the kitchen, thanking her, and she leaves.

You are back in the living room, but that cake haunts you. You decide to have "just one slice." (Hah!) You imagine that you arise, go back into the kitchen, and get a plate and a knife. You see yourself cutting into the delicious cake. Just then swarms of ants and cockroaches run out of the cake. You end your relaxation.

Just reading this, it may be a long time before you enjoy another piece of chocolate cake. But when you relax and picture in this way, your mind receives instructions that make chocolate cake absolutely detestable to you.

You can devise obnoxious techniques for any problem food.

For problem thoughts, there are "switch" techniques that work just as powerfully. You can instruct your mind that every time you think of eating when you are not really hungry, your appetite will disappear if you take a drink of cold water.

Do you keep cold water in the refrigerator? If so, this is a good "switch" for you to use. Relax, imagine, then use the following words and their picture counterpart:

Words—"Whenever false hunger occurs between meals—and since I am eating two extra mini-meals, all such hunger is false—then all I need to do is drink some cold water and the appetite will disappear."

Picture—See yourself heading for food in between meals. Then, instead of eating, visualize yourself reaching for cold water, pouring it, then going back to what you were doing before, with no desire to

Accelerating a New Attractive Look

eat. Also, picture yourself abstaining from and eliminating excess food between meals.

You can use this substitution technique for anything and with anything. False hunger responds easily. Some of the substitutes that you can instruct your mind to accept in its place are:

Three deep breaths

A brisk walk

A stalk of celery

A book

But water is at the top of my list. We need water. It fills the stomach temporarily. It is refreshing and restoring. It merits our confidence.

One Day At A Time Adds Up to Several Pounds Lost

When you gain weight, you do it one day at a time. You do not set foolish goals: "I want to be a fatty by next Easter."

Pounds need to be eliminated this same way—one day at a time. My plan works exactly in this way. You go day by day. You are now approaching the end of this book. So the One Day may be tomorrow, or the next day.

You enjoy each One Day. You do not think about the next day. You merely experience the One Day now—today.

Later, you experience the next day. It is not important to be aware that you are consciously repeating the One Day. It is *extremely important* that you eat whatever you know is correct; that you think positive, desirable, loving thoughts today—this One Day.

Hopefully, you will have studied the allowed and nonallowed food lists in "ME." Hopefully, you will have written about yourself in "ME" and instructed your mind to eat, think, and do correctly.

If so, then let your life unfold one day at a time. No pushing for fast but self-defeating weight loss. No setting unreasonable time limits. No anxiety. No tumult. No trying. No willpower. No rationalizations. No excuses. No fear. No failure.

You acquire a philosophical attitude about your weight. For example, Sandra O., who at age 32, height five feet eight inches, was only 5 pounds away from reaching 300.

Sandra did quite well. She lost 60 pounds in five months.

Then her loss stopped and she communicated this to me:

"I'm afraid of losing more weight. I reach a certain point, then this wall appears and I don't want to go any further. Logically thinking, there is nothing from the past that can hurt me and I shouldn't have to worry about it. It's kinda like when I reach a certain point, everything from the past catches up with me. I shouldn't worry about such things as I can't change them anyway. The events and negative feelings of the past prevent me from going forward. My greatest problem is that I don't love me. Sometimes I even hate me."

Recording it on paper meant self-enlightenment, then her weight loss resumed. That prompted her to write again about a new, positive, uplifting attitude:

"I don't feel as though I'm on a diet anymore; just eating sensibly and learning more about *me* one day at a time. I no longer think about how much weight I have shed other than when I weigh in at the time of my appointments. I just think about the program, doing and un-doing one day at a time—a completely new attitude about me and my weight problem. If I looked at all the excess weight I had to lose every day, I know I would 'blow it.' If I thought about it, I'd drown in such thoughts.

"The One Day At A Time Approach has been a tremendous help. If I thought much about what I've already done (looking back complacently), I'd be tempted to backslide. If I looked at all the weight I still had to lose, it would overwhelm me and I'd 'blow it.' So, I just think what my final weight goal and programming is all about and know that I will reach it sometime in the future—no set date—success will come eventually with lots of work and patience; it's what I think, do and undo one day at a time that really counts!

"I have my little picture of how I'm going to look and be in the back of my mind. When the going gets rough and I'm desperate, I bring that picture to the fore-front of my mind—it helps a lot. Over the week-end I had a terrible craving for sweets. In the past I used to stuff myself with angel food cake and I would 'blow it.' I thought about the reason: My husband was angry with me and I wanted affection. When my spouse is affectionate to me, he is sweet to me. This time though, I chewed gum, sat down and wrote some letters, wrote about my feelings and attitudes. The urge eventually passed. It was almost like—if I couldn't get affection, then this did the trick instead! Seems as though I'm learning and helping myself more and more—one day at a time."

XI

SMALLER PORTIONS WITH A GREATER, ENJOYABLE TASTE

There is a physician who has perfected a device for smokers. Although production has been limited, it has proven to be effective in limiting cigarette consumption. It is a combination lighter, clip, and container. The smoker uses it to light up, then after a deep drag or two on the cigarette, he clips off the burning end and stores the remainder of the cigarette for later use.

The device materially reduces cigarette consumption, since most smokers obtain their greatest satisfaction from lighting up and taking that first puff.

The same is true about food. We often obtain more satisfaction from the dinner event than we do from eating the food itself. Suppose you were informed, "No dinner tonight." It gives you an immediate sense of panic. On the other hand, "Dinner will be at seven" gives you an immediate sense of warmth and security. It often is unimportant what food is being served; just that dinner is being served.

Take the cigarette smoker. If there is an urge to smoke, but an interruption takes place—no problem. The cigarette waits. On the other hand, if there is an urge to smoke, but there are no cigarettes on hand, everything else waits until the package is obtained.

My patients cut portions in half and do not consider that they are eating half portions. They are extracting a full measure of enjoyment from the smaller portions, because most of the enjoyment comes from the eating event and from those first few savory mouthfuls of each food item. Quality of food is important.

Since there are now two more eating events, thanks to the "Rule of Two," the total eating enjoyment for the day on the One-Day-At-A-Time Plan is increased and intensified.

Half portions + 2 extra meals = more enjoyment, more "kiks." It also equals less fuel for the body's "furnace" and a conversion of weight gain to weight loss.

There is no standard portion. There is no gauge either in weight or volume that defines whether a portion is not enough or too much. Adjust daily food intake as necessary in order to eliminate plateaus and keep the pounds rolling off. Quantity of food is important.

In Japan, portions are generally tiny by American standards. In Germany, portions are generally immense by American standards.

A "standard portion" is the quantity of food we have become used to. One family may eat portions that are quite different in size from another family's portions. One restaurant may serve materially larger portions than another.

There is an all-you-can-eat for $3.99 buffet restaurant that hides the dinner plates on a lower shelf but keeps the smaller salad plates within easy reach. People use the smaller salad plates. Although they pile them high and the patrons eat all they desire, the restaurant comes out ahead.

The stomach does not have to be full in order for you to have a "full feeling." Chances are that the "full feeling" you have experienced in the past is an "overfull feeling." You were literally stuffed. Your portions were oversized.

In this chapter we will study the anatomy of "full" and I will show you ways to cut your portions in half almost without knowing the difference. Smaller size portions make a smaller sized you.

How to Make a Smaller Portion Just As Filling

There are two people eating, each in his own home. Let us eavesdrop and see who is eating larger portions.

John is a gourmet. He had prepared baked veal chops for himself. He sliced carrots and celery and placed them at the bottom of a casserole. He sprinkled a little thyme over them and placed four veal chops, each an inch thick, on top. A little salt substitute and pepper with just enough water to cover the vegetables, and the casserole was ready for the oven, already preheated to 375 degrees.

John read his evening paper for an hour. Now he was ready for the baked veal chops and they were browned and ready for him. He prepared his salad in a separate bowl and carried it and the baking dish to the table. He looked at it. Just right. He placed one of the chops on his dinner plate, along with the bed of vegetables. It had a tempting aroma. He dug in. Chewing slowly, he marveled at his own skill. The chops were deliciously flavored by a mixture of their own juices and the vegetable juices. Next time he might include a slice or two of onion.

Carolyn, a block away, had returned from an exasperating day at the office. Aside from this, her divorced husband was two weeks late in the monthly alimony payment. She hated to call him. It was always such a hassle. She took the pot of leftover beef stew from yesterday and heated it. While she waited, an imaginary conversation with her ex heated and boiled in her mind.

She brought the pot to the table, served herself, and began to eat. He'll play on my sympathy like last time, she thought. If that doesn't work he'll want to come over to see me, seeking to get us to try again. That could easily lead to a beating and another trip to the hospital for me.

Carolyn reached for some more stew. There was none.

Who ate the larger portion? Who was more relaxed and at ease?

When John finished his one veal chop and his salad, he carried the casserole with the three remaining chops into the kitchen, covered it, and placed it in the refrigerator. Maybe he would have another chop later with a cup of tea.

Carolyn reached for more stew without realizing that she had already taken a second and a third portion. There was none left.

Carolyn ate far more than John. But it was automatic, impulsive eating. She actually did not realize how much she was eating. She derived no "kiks" from her food as she went through the motions of eating.

John, on the other hand, savored every delicious bite. He appreciated his handiwork. He derived "kiks" from his food.

The key to obtaining more "mileage" out of smaller portions is *awareness of enjoyment*.

If your mind wanders while you are eating, you are missing "kiks." Since you basically require "kiks," missed "kiks" necessitate more food.

Talking while you eat creates the desire for larger portions. Worrying while you eat creates the desire for larger portions. Not paying attention to your food while you eat creates the desire for larger portions. Extraneous activities while you eat create the desire for larger portions. This usually creates a larger you.

Become aware of the food on your fork as it enters your mouth. Become aware of its taste. Become aware of its texture. Become aware of its "kiks." Food awareness magnifies the satisfaction value of your portions and minimizes your weight.

It does not matter how large a portion you take. If you are not aware of eating it, you are a candidate for a second portion—or a third—or a fourth. Develop your awareness—learn to think. Don't eat impulsively (compulsively?). Think before and while eating.

As Jane D., 24, became more aware of eating every bite, she discovered an awareness of every bite of life, too. "I have been going to the beach now," she told me. "I experience and enjoy nature day by day. A stroll in the park is now an important event. I enjoy reading more than I used to. I started guitar lessons. I communicate better with my husband because I am now an aware listener."

Jane went from 164 to 136 in three aware months.

When you pay attention, smaller portions are much more filling and satisfying than large portions.

Other Techniques for Losing Weight with Smaller Portions

Awareness is the key.

But awareness can be interfered with by "static." The environment is creating sounds, sights, smells, and touch sensations. These can overwhelm, cloud, even obliterate a more subtle input—taste.

There is a restaurant in New England that has no name. It is located in a gracious home with a subdued atmosphere. You would pass it by if you did not see a small sign at the driveway saying, "Serving the Evening Meal."

Is the food good? You bet it is. But I will wager that the very same food served at a drive-in alongside of a Los Angeles freeway would not taste the same. Certainly it would not be as enjoyable.

You need a subdued place in your home in which to enjoy your meals. Perhaps candlelight. Soft music. A simple arrangement of flowers. And quiet conversation.

Eating alone is no excuse for not eating graciously. The tendency is to prepare what is easiest, nothing special, and eat it watching television or reading. Set a respectable table for yourself. Use your best silver. Spend time to prepare a dinner worthy of you. Then enjoy it leisurely, knowing you are in good company—the best.

You should not permit family conversation at your dinner table of a combative or defensive nature. Dinner conversation should be small talk. It should be pleasant, interesting, and positive.

The spotlight should be on food.

Every bite deserves your full attention. No food slips down your gullet unnoticed. You derive more enjoyment from a smaller portion when each forkful is a taste celebration than from larger portions which are wolfed down.

Since you will be chewing longer and eating in slow motion as I have already advised, there will be longer periods of silence at the table. To those accustomed to constant chatter, this may seem awkward. But you will find that quiet moments together are memorable moments. You may even remember how delicious the salmon tasted that evening.

You may think what I say next is obvious, but . . .

Here's a weight clincher: *leave something on your plate.*

"Hold it," you say, "That makes a smaller portion even smaller."

Yes, but something else happens, something that is not obvious. Remember, there is nothing about the size of a portion that makes it large or small, just habit. When a portion is larger than we are used to, we generally leave some. Leaving something on the plate then is connected in our "programmed" mind to sufficiency. Thus, when you leave even one forkful on your plate, you are instructing your mind to accept whatever you have eaten as sufficient.

It has another advantage. Most of us have been taught since early childhood to clean our plates. "Finish your dinner, or you won't get dessert." Or, "finish your cereal; think of all the starving people in China." Just what good your clean plate will do for starving people anywhere is doubtful, but we persist in saying that to our children, who probably know better than we do when they have had enough.

You do not *have to* clean your plate. You do not *have to* leave something on your plate, either. But you may find that leaving, instead of cleaning, makes smaller portions appear larger.

Lose with Smaller Portions of This, Larger Portions of That

Some allowable foods also contain fat or carbohydrates. A balanced, nutritious intake is essential. However, should your weight loss reach a plateau where that needle on the scale refuses to budge day after day, don't become discouraged. *Don't discourage yourself.* Don't rationalize or allow yourself to backslide and fail.

Discouragement is fattening.

You are in control. Learn to control.

Examine the allowable foods again. Note there are some foods allowed in moderation or with some caution.

Fruit is an item that requires caution. Slow down on fruit. You are permitted to have fruit once a day. Perhaps once a day may be too much, especially if you are eating a large piece of fruit, such as a huge peach or pear or a large portion of melon or berries. Once a day may also be too much if you are eating the wrong fruits with large amounts of fruit sugar, such as oranges, apples, bananas, grapes, raisins, or fruits canned in syrup.

You can start the needle of the scale moving down again by substituting a lean hamburger patty for a pear, or a shrimp cocktail for a peach, or —— for a ——.

You then need to look at your vegetable consumption. Are you letting green peas slip into your menus? Or potatoes? Or yams? Or lima beans? Or beets? These are "No-Nos." There are plenty of delicious vegetables on the allowable list. They are on the list because they are low in starch. Some, such as broccoli, are not only low in starch but also higher than most vegetables and grains in protein. There is more protein in a stalk of broccoli than in a slice of whole-wheat bread.

The key to selecting vegetables is *the pulp.* Beans have varying amounts of pulp. A string bean has the least, so it is allowed. However, the large thick variety of bean such as the lima bean, is to be avoided. Corn, rice, and all but the green squashes are practically pure starch.

Search your menus for other carbohydrates that can be cut. Is sugar or flour sneaking in somewhere? Whack! Chop off starch wherever it rears its fattening head.

Fat is next. Fats and oils creep into many menus. Cut down, cut out. Use coated pans that permit you to cook without oil. Avoid butter, margarine, sweet and sour cream (also half and half). Flavored yogurt is fattening because it is sweetened. Nuts have fat. Avocado has fat.

Be more conscientious about trimming away fat in meat and poultry, eating around it, and removing poultry skin.

Exclude thickened soups and gravies. When you dine out, request that salt be omitted. Don't accept a baked potato just because "it comes with the dinner." Insist on a substitution. "Sliced tomatoes instead, please." Skip restaurants that are not cooperative in this regard. There are many that are.

If you do have to cut down sharply on fruits and vegetables to get the weight progress going again, you should be taking vitamin and mineral supplements. Obtain the roughage your body needs by eating plenty of raw salad.

Roughage or fiber keeps your colon functioning and helps your body to eliminate waste products. Water does this, too. So, remember your eight glasses of water or equivalent each day.

Although you cut down sharply on fat and oil, there is enough in the allowable foods to satisfy your body's needs. Traces of fat and oil are all we need. The low-calorie dressing you are using on your salad will supply your oil requirements.

Sights and Sounds That Trigger False Hunger

You are enjoying smaller portions, two extra meals, high-protein foods, writing about your feelings, and instructing your mind to move you to a happier, healthier, more enlightened and slender self.

But the world is the same. Your family is there. The television programs are the same. The supermarkets have the same foods. Your job is still from 9 to 5, and in the same place, doing the same thing.

The environment that instructed your mind since birth is still there, still molding you in the way it did before, still ungainfully influencing you toward gaining weight.

Someone in the family, while clearing the table, munches on a leftover. A dish of cookies is placed near the couch. Magazines show cake embellished with icing in their full-colored ads. The television commercials make white bread seem good for you.

Supermarket shelves are bulging with sweet delights that reach out to you by dint of psychologically designed packages—enemies in disguise. Candy machines and coke machines and pastry machines dot office buildings along with fast, fatty food outlets. There is no let-up. You are fair game. You are the prey and the hunters never lay down their weapons.

This molding process is pretty strong stuff. It is instructing your mind constantly whereas you are relaxing and giving yourself countermanding instructions only once or twice a day; that is, if you remember.

Countermanding instructions must be given frequently and implicitly. Also, you need to take countermeasures. The countermeasures must be "strong stuff," too.

The countermeasures can be of two types—defensive or offensive.

Defensive measures imply reducing your exposure to the external forces that pressure you to eat fattening foods and to overeat. Some examples:

Don't permit nonallowed snacks in your house.

Eat in only one place in your home.

Adhere to your shopping list when in the supermarket.

Don't read food ads.

Look away during food commercials.

Use affirmatives like "Not for me!"

Avoid restaurants that feature fat, starch, or sugar.

Travel by routes that minimize restaurant sights.

Change the subject, if about food.

Wash, or dry, but let others clean the before- and after-meal dishes and store the food.

Attack measures include:

Speak out against and eliminate white sugar and white flour from your food intake.

Patronize health food stores or low-calorie dietetic sections at the market.

Be a "missionary" for the One-Day-At-A-Time Plan.

Use more relaxation and mental "instruction" sessions.

Write in "ME" on this subject to see what other slenderizing attack measures surface.

Smaller Portions of Quality Protein Are Larger Portions of Nourishment

This whole idea of smaller portions appears restrictive to many of my patients—until they apply it to themselves.

It may seem restrictive to you now, just reading about it.

In a nonrestrictive one day of correct and enjoyable food intake such as this which does not require you to count calories; which does not ask you to cut out foods—merely to switch foods; and which does not even ask you to continue with it more than a day; cutting portions in half may seem drastic.

Nonetheless, when you embark on this program, you will find it to be a "natural." Smaller portions may be all you really need for several reasons:

1. You have added two meals (mini-meals); thus you are eating more often to compensate for the smaller portions.

2. The time between meals is decreased.

3. You are eating fewer carbohydrates, which tend to leave your stomach rapidly, leaving you with an empty feeling.

4. You are eating more protein, which takes longer to digest; thus you retain the full feeling longer with smaller portions.

The more protein, at the expense of carbohydrates, the less weight. Of course, you need some carbohydrates for their vitamins, minerals, and roughage. They also help keep a correct acid-alkaline balance. But if you are taking vitamin and mineral supplements, and if you are drinking eight glasses of fluid daily, which is an integral part of this program, you are minimizing any chance of acidity or mineral-vitamin deficiency, even with a menu of only 10 percent carbohydrates.

There is no possible problem of too much protein, especially if you are enjoying diversified sources. Minimum daily requirements have been set as two ounces (56 grams) for men, and 1.6 ounces (45 grams) for women.

The proteins we are most likely to eat—the animal proteins—are the easiest for the body to utilize in the vital processes. Quality proteins are beef, veal, lamb, poultry, and fish. Milk, eggs, and cheese also provide complete or high-quality protein.

There is some incomplete protein in whole-grain cereals, beans, and corn. But you extract more benefit from smaller portions of milk and eggs in comparison to beans and cereals because of the complete proteins found in these products. This spells more nourishment, less weight—a most important consideration in your weight-loss plan.

Your body knows this, so it gives you the "satisfied" signal with smaller portions. And your mind is equally satisfied.

Instruct Your Mind to Make Smaller Portions Appear Larger

You can use your mental instructions to help adjust to smaller portions. And smaller portions equal a smaller you.

All of the words and pictures you have been given in the previous chapters are in reality "wish actualizers." The mental words and pictures are not only instructions to the mind, they are downright commands.

This phenomenal brain of ours obeys, even if we are giving "impossible" orders.

Your orders can make cold seem hot and will even produce a simulated blister.

They can distort time and can make the time in between meals seem like minutes instead of hours.

They can distort taste and can make favorite foods taste horrible.

It is a simple matter to give your mind instructions to see smaller portions as no longer small.

The deeper you are relaxed, the better these distortion-creating instructions take hold. However, you cannot just begin with a distortion-creating instruction. First, you need to practice your relaxing and self-instructing techniques by using easier, positive types of words and clear mental images. Then, if you have to use distortion later, it works for you.

For instance, this is fine:

Words—"I am satisfied with smaller portions."

Picture—See yourself with a smaller plate and being just as satisfied.

But this should be used only if reinforcement is needed.

Words—"These portions are large. I see them as large and am satisfied by them."

Picture—See yourself smaller in size at the table, with everything relatively larger.

Relaxing and imagining (creating mental pictures) is powerful stuff. Use it. But use it creatively and positively. Use it to help you love yourself, to eat healthfully, and to continue with the program, one day at a time.

Some call it daydreaming. Some call it meditation. Some call it self-hypnosis. But whatever you call it, it is still *you* straightening out *you*—learning to understand and to do for yourself. Straightening yourself out results in weight loss.

You Can Snack on the One-Day-At-A-Time Plan

There are many misconceptions about being overweight. Overweight people have something wrong with their glands. Not necessarily true. Overweight people are gluttons. Not true. Obesity is inherited. Not true.

What is true: overweight people eat the wrong foods. They also eat when they are "triggered" by false hunger (appetite).

Switch wrong foods to right foods, remove the emotional connection to the mental appetite (false hunger) stimulants, and the problem is solved—permanently.

You can eat generous amounts of some foods and still lose weight. You can snack between meals—on the right foods (pages 47–9). However, smaller portions are prescribed in this program because of the two extra mini-meals ("Rule of Two") plus the necessity to achieve your desired weight.

Right now, before you start this program, you are probably not eating too much food. But you are, without a shadow of a doubt, eating the wrong foods.

So don't get "hung-up" by this idea of smaller portions. It is a natural outcome of the changes you are making. Your body will be supplied with more real food on the One-Day-At-A-Time Plan than it is now receiving. And, amazingly, you will continue to shed the excess fat.

Eating correctly allows for larger portions of certain foods on that One Day. Liberal snacking is permissible with certain foods, such as unlimited vegetables.

You can always have a slice of lean meat. You can always have some low-fat cottage cheese. You can always have leftover greens such as spinach, turnip tops, beet tops, dandelion greens, taro tops, and of course salad materials such as lettuce, cucumbers, carrot sticks, celery, or watercress.

When you "raid" the refrigerator, besides the above snacks, you can always have a leftover piece of fish or a chicken leg (skin removed). You can always have a few mushrooms, broiled or raw, a hard-boiled egg, or a slice of cheese. Become more considerate about the food stored in your refrigerator. It will return the compliment—in pounds off.

Cooked rhubarb, a vegetable often used as a dessert "fruit," is a good snack. It needs no sugar. The tangy flavor is refreshing and it does not count in your allowable daily fruit intake.

Some Alternatives to the One-Day Plan

Permissiveness is the key to the success of the One-Day-At-A-Time Plan. *Enjoyment* of new eating and thinking habits is its secret. *And a new self-image is its insurance.*

You do not pay a price to go on the One-Day Plan. Instead, you receive a bonus. The bonus you receive is in food enjoyment, a slimmer contour, peace of mind, and a boosted level of health.

There are some alternatives. But the price you pay can be exorbitant. For example: Behavior modification in a clinic or group situation involves sharing your personal problems. It, too, involves a journal or book but requires blocks of time over an extended period. If modification of thought is given a secondary role, the weight problem will eventually return. Extra pounds "cost" you a heavy price.

Another example is fasting. Fasting can be a traumatic experience. Long-term fasting, usually averaging three to four weeks, can bring physical and mental duress. This is minimized with short-term fasting, usually 10 to 14 days. But not eating for this length of time is a rough price to pay for weight lost that you'll probably regain sooner or later—*especially* if you have not given yourself the mental instructions to lose the fat between the ears—one day at a time.

Then there is calorie counting. Counting calories can be made easy with calorie-counters, but somehow food has a way of slipping past without being counted. Whenever this happens, you slip, backslide, then regain the lost weight.

The protein-sparing liquid *diet* has been declared dangerous. I have already commented on the damaging effect this can have, especially if it is not supervised by your physician or bariatrician.

Dieting and diets per se *cannot* resolve the overweight problem. They are hopelessly and ultimately self-defeating. Dieting is an endless exercise of frustration and eventual failure. A diet or gimmick *cannot* solve the problem—you.

There are no alternatives to thinking, understanding, enjoying, and doing for yourself. There are no satisfying or successful alternatives to this One-Day-At-A-Time Weight-Loss Plan.

XII

THE FIRST DAY OF THE REST OF YOUR FOREVER SLENDER LIFE

What are you having for dinner tomorrow night?

How about baked burgers Vienna style? These are lean meat patties shaped around slices of hard-boiled eggs. How about slicing some mushrooms and combining with zucchini for a special gourmet salad? This delightful repast could be your dinner on the one day of correct, improved, and enjoyable eating.

Or how about tomato juice, veal steak with green peppers, a bran muffin, and buttermilk?

Or how about a broiled minute steak with onions, cherry tomatoes, and green pepper strips? Some blueberries for dessert? If you have roast lamb the next day with green asparagus, mixed salad, and cold rhubarb, you have repeated the one day of improved food intake.

Frankly, it is going to be difficult for you to get off the one day of correct eating. You won't be playing the "On-Off Game" any longer. It will mean more fun, energy and attractiveness to go on . . . and on.

Do you see now why I asked that you read this book before beginning? Let's sum up. You already know much more about yourself than you did when you originally opened this book. You know more about food, portions, and how to instruct your mind. You have and know more about a plan—your One-Day-At-A-Time Weight-Loss Plan.

And you know the best part: it has all been so effortless, effective, satisfying, slenderizing, and beautifying.

All this change and new planning is about to happen. What this final chapter says is, "Get ready, get set—go!"

The Reward System for Changing Eating Habits

Behavior therapy programs developed for obesity problems frequently entail a system of rewards. One popular system is like the gold stars we used to earn in elementary school, only instead of the gummed paper stars, the client is given a certificate indicating that a number of points have been earned for a new, learned behavior.

For instance, a client reports that he or she went to a party and ate celery and cheese dip instead of sandwiches. "Congratulations, you are awarded ten points." Later, these points are converted into a prize of some kind—a gift certificate for new clothes, a trip to Disneyland, or the like.

These rewards act as reinforcement to the new behavior.

I believe in the reward system. You work. You are paid.

However, the One-Day-At-A-Time Plan has been designed to be its own reward. It is therefore its own reinforcement. It flows naturally, and this is as it should be. Fantastic!

What are its rewards? Here are ten. They are more rewarding than ten points or ten stars:

No stringent curtailments, so no test of illogical, self-deceptive willpower. No trying. You flow with it.

Good food, even gourmet food, with emphasis on eating fun.

Shorter intervals between meals, because you are rewarded with two extra mini-meals.

Improved nourishment due to proteins, minerals, and vitamins, which means you are rewarded with a higher level of bodily well-being and improved health.

Elimination improves due to fluids and roughage. You feel and become lighter, more buoyant.

Increased energy supply all day due to the lasting power of protein.

Feeling of exhilaration as you lose weight effortlessly, successfully, with no more need for debasing self-incrimination, self-failure, and self-hate.

Insight and understanding about yourself as you write, leading to self-understanding, self-mastery, and self-love. Also, leading to your ultimate weight goal.

Heightened self-concept and self-image resulting from mental instructions with rewards extending to sexual, social, economic, and many other benefits.

A normalizing in weight resulting in a longevity bonus and personal happiness as the excess pounds melt away.

Which would you rather have—free tickets to a show, ten stars, or these ten "rewards"?

These are not the only rewards of the One-Day-At-A-Time Plan. Each of these ten are like pebbles thrown into a lake. The ripples keep extending out into your life, day after day, year after year. When you receive rewards like these, you don't need willpower.

Believe my thousands of slenderized patients—the rewards are endless, the miracles fathomless, the happiness supreme.

Have you found one paragraph in this book where I exhort you to use willpower? "You must be committed to accepting responsibility for strength or weakness. You must resolve to put temptation behind you. You must try harder if you are to succeed!"

Hogwash!

The harder you try, the sooner you will fail.

A program must develop, flow, and come easily. It must be more rewarding than a sugary taste or quick and easy.

Compare the rewards of sugar and flour to the rewards I enumerated above. Comparing intellectually is only the beginning. Experiencing them day after day, beginning tomorrow, is the real reward.

As I said before, once you begin the One-Day program, you will need willpower to get off. And willpower fails. If you don't think so, remember your past diets. And look at your overweight friends.

You Talk About Being Born Again

"It is really great. It has a snowballing effect. I eat and think sensibly, naturally. For the first time in my life, I love me."

"I have switched from desserts to desert. Whenever things become impossible at home, instead of eating, I spend a day or two away at a desert resort. It is a better tonic than dessert. I am pulling my life and myself together."

"As an airline stewardess, people dump their troubles on me. But, needing love and affection, too, I turn to sweets and junk foods. Now, I know what I have been doing—short circuiting my feelings. I've adjusted my automatic pilot for positive reactions, one day at a time. I am feeling beautiful again."

These three patients all write of their transformation in different ways. Yet it all adds up to one common denominator—a new life style, a new life, a new you—a miracle.

What they are saying is, "I have been born again."

For each person, the unwanted "old" that drops away is different. Dorothy H. lists ten changes derived from having been on the One-Day-At-A-Time Plan:

"1. I'm using my mental 'instructions' for cigarettes and liquor as well as food, *and it works.*

2. I don't feel deprived or a martyr.

3. I was living to eat, now I eat to live.

4. I sleep better than I have for years—a miracle.

5. My longstanding ulcer is improved (X-rays confirm)—another miracle.

6. I'm losing inches as well as pounds, from a slack size 18 to size 12 in no time.

7. I *shop* at the supermarket instead of *buy.*

8. I am thinking of and for myself for the first time in years.

9. I adopt mental 'instructions' as an everyday way to change my life.

10. I think and write about myself, enjoying it, as the pounds fall off."

Charles D., a student of Zen, enjoys the mental instructions as they fit into his scheme of things:

"I see myself pounds lighter. I see myself eating only that which is good for my body and mind. I see myself as in the 'circle and the point,' a part of the natural order of things, united in body and mind, purified in spirit."

You are not Dorothy H. Nor are you Charles D. You are a unique person.

What you write will be different.

What you think will be different.

What you eat will be different.

What you say and do will be different.

What you experience in the Plan will be different.

But it will all add up to the same thing—a great new life, a great new YOU.

Fear of Failure Is Fattening

As tomorrow draws near, know that all past failures are due to diets that are restrictive, boring, unrealistic, and eventually self-defeating. This plan is not. You *cannot* fail. I mention this because any fear of failure can work against you—*only* if you allow it.

If you have been on the diet "yo-yo," losing and gaining back weight time and time again, it is natural for you to have a sense of impending failure. You have learned to fail all by yourself.

This is a thought habit due to repeated mental conditioning. You think failure now out of habit. It is a habit you have etched into your subconsciousness by repeated, negative mental instructions. It is a false thought and an undesirable habit. This program is different. It eliminates past failure-oriented factors.

These failure factors include willpower, setting false and unrealistic goals, losing weight rapidly, trying, lack of self-understanding, plus others mentioned in preceding chapters.

I offer you *no* chance to fail. I offer you only the opportunity to succeed.

Fear of failure is as fattening as guilt, loneliness, rejection, and other negative "put-downs."

Anna S., 48, had an intense, prolonged struggle with her weight and her fear of failure:

"I want to dare to try to be a fine artist. I want to dare to live each day to the fullest. I want to dare to be truly alive each waking moment. That's living.

"But I have been hiding. I have been afraid. Afraid of what? As a child I was afraid of a spanking. Now what? I don't know, but I feel I am full of fears I don't even know about. I see them in my conversation. I use words that betray my fears. I'm chicken. I'm afraid to fail."

Not long after writing this, Anna eliminated these fears through fearless instructions. She relaxed, said positive words, visualized positive pictures, performed the activities in her notebook ("ME"), and the false fears dissolved along with some 30 pounds of unwanted fat.

Andrea W. gained insight into the reason for her 170 pounds on a five foot five frame, but not until she went on this One-Day-At-A-Time program at the age of 47.

"It's the fear of failure," she told me. "If I succeed I won't have any excuse for failing. I really fear success, not failure! Success is unknown, unfamiliar—it's uncomfortable. I have been sabotaging success all my life. Now that I realize this, I'm eliminating failure patterns one day at a time. Success is becoming more familiar to me. I am beginning to like the taste of it."

Often, fears lurk deep within our mind and are difficult to identify. The words we use often help to identify those deep fears and dark thoughts, especially fear of failure.

Here are some:

I wasn't cut out for success. I'm a born failure.
Fate has dealt me a cruel blow. My luck ran out.
Food is my downfall. Temptation got the better of me.
I was born with two strikes against me. Life's impossible.
Misery loves company. I'm fat, I'm happy.
There's just no way out. I'm in a rut.
I'm tired all the time. I have tired blood.
You just don't change overnight. It takes a long time.
I'm a compulsive eater. I'm frustrated.
I'm a creature of habit. I've been programmed.
I've been overweight for years. It's my destiny.
It's hard to control myself. I can't help it.
It's impossible. The problem is overwhelming.
I am stymied. I can't understand what it's all about.
This is getting me down. I'm a depressed person.
I could care less. I have no desire.
It's getting harder to get ahead. I don't have enough time.
I find it doesn't help. I haven't got a chance.
It's hard to break the habit. I'll quit eating.
I'm a weak person. I don't have enough willpower.
It's no use. I tried, didn't I?
It's hopeless. There's no future.
I have an inferiority complex. I'm a negative person.
You're thin, I'm obese. I lost the battle of the bulge.
It just wasn't meant to be. What will be will be.

It's too late. Success is not for me.
I'm absent-minded. It slipped my mind.
I can't help myself. I have a tendency to be fat.
I feel so guilty and ashamed. I'll have a cookie and feel better.
You can't teach an old dog new tricks. It's hard to learn.
He can but I can't. I really don't know why I'm this way.
Life is passing me by. Woe is me, I know I'll fail.
I don't think. I'm confused and mixed up.
I couldn't refuse and hurt her feelings. I'll sacrifice.
I let myself down. I "blew it."
My nerves got the better of me. I'm a nervous person.
I'm afraid of failing. I'm afraid of success.
Do any of these strike a resonant chord in you?
Then mentally think "Cancel." Turn the words and thoughts around. Turn yourself (your head) around.

Give yourself a boost with correct, positive words to replace these failure words. Give yourself a boost with the correct, positive, slenderizing thoughts to replace these failure thoughts.

A Special "Accelerator" for Rapid Weight Loss

There are many overweight people who may be viewing the One-Day-At-A-Time Plan as a prolonged period of slow weight loss. This is not the reason why I say to be patient and not set week-to-week or month-to-month goals; unrealistic, limiting, and self-defeating goals.

The reason I ask you to avoid these goals is that they are stress factors. You and I want to eliminate both physical and mental stress, not add to it.

There are ways, as I explained in Chapter X, of accelerating weight loss. But, to prove that I am not endorsing slow progress as opposed to fast progress, I am now going to give you an "accelerator" for this program.

It is not mandatory.
It is optional.
It is beneficial and helpful.
It is a weight-loss "accelerator."

It involves the liquid protein that I have already discussed. Remember, I said you can use it as one of your daily meals. Well, you can increase this within certain limits. These limits are prescribed below with options. I am spelling this out very carefully, but you should still do this under your physician's or bariatrician's supervision.

Protein Supplemental Plans

Directions: Below are six *optional* protein supplemental plans. *Use only one plan at a time* as an aid in your weight-control program.

The predigested protein liquid may be taken undiluted (See NOTE on page 213).

Daily

1. Drink one 8-ounce glass of prepared (see directions below), predigested protein as a substitute for one meal.
2. Drink one 4-ounce glass of prepared, predigested protein as a substitute for one meal and one 4-ounce glass of protein mid-morning or mid-afternoon.

Every Third Day

3. Drink one 8-ounce glass of prepared (see directions below), predigested protein as a substitute for breakfast and one as a substitute for lunch.
4. Drink one 4-ounce glass of prepared, predigested protein as a substitute for breakfast and one as a substitute for lunch. Also, drink one 4-ounce glass of predigested protein mid-morning and mid-afternoon.

Every Fourth Day

5. Drink one 8-ounce glass of prepared (see directions below), predigested protein as a substitute for each one of your three meals.
6. Drink one 4-ounce glass of prepared, predigested protein as a substitute for each of your three meals. Also drink one 4-ounce glass of predigested protein mid-morning, mid-afternoon, and evening.

Preparation of the Liquid Predigested Protein Drink

To 2 tablespoons (1 ounce) of predigested protein liquid add one of the following: 7 ounces of ice water (with a wedge of lemon or lime), 7 ounces of club soda, 7 ounces of diet soda, 7 ounces of non-fat or skim milk. Stir well and add ice cubes. Artificial flavoring (extract) or fresh fruit (from the low-carbohydrate list) may be added sparingly for variety. You may wish to mix contents in a blender with crushed ice. Sip the drink slowly, allowing your taste buds to savor its delicious taste. This in turn will produce a feeling of fullness and satisfaction.

NOTE: If desired, you may take 2 tablespoons of undiluted, predigested liquid protein; then follow with 7 ounces or less of ice water, diet soda, tea or coffee, etc.

Preparation of the Powder Predigested Protein Drink

To 2 talespoons of unflavored, predigested protein powder add 8 ounces of non-fat or skim milk. Add artificial sweetener (liquid or powder) or artificial flavoring (extract) or fresh fruit sparingly to taste. The fresh fruit from the low-carbohydrate list is preferred. You may use unsweetened fruit juice, water-packed, dietetic, or diabetic canned fruit sparingly to taste. Mix in a blender for one minute. Add ice cubes or crushed ice and mix again for one minute. Different combinations of flavoring will allow variety. Sip slowly and enjoy your protein cocktail.

Permitted on All Liquid Predigested Protein Days (every fourth day)

Water, hot or iced coffee or tea (decaffeinated preferred), 8 ounces of tomato juice or V-8 juice, Bloody Mary mix (without liquor), diet soda, club soda (with a wedge of lemon or lime), clear broth bouillon. Also, unlimited, low-starch vegetables (see list) are permitted.

NOTE: Avoid the exclusive use of predigested protein liquid or powder as it could result in untoward side effects and problems—*follow only one of the plans outlined above*. Although these plans are optional, nevertheless, they can help you to achieve and maintain your desired weight. Be sure to take daily vitamin and mineral supplements as recommended by your family physician. A predigested protein soup mix may be occasionally substituted for the predigested protein drink. If necessary, a small quantity of natural, unprocessed bran flakes or granules may be included in the blend to help maintain proper elimination.

A Final Word About Weighty Problems

As you prepare to embark on the One-Day-At-A-Time Plan, I want to say a final word about problems.

We all have problems. Yet, some of us are slender, others are overweight. What makes the difference is how we react to those problems. What makes the difference is how you react to yourself as *you* confront your day-to-day problems and situations. This is attitude. It helps to mold our emotions, feelings, and life style.

We can have or develop an attitude of defeat and pessimism. Then the problem becomes weighty, and you become overweight. Or, we can have and develop an attitude of "This, too, will pass." Then the problem is not weighty and you achieve normal weight.

You think you have problems? Listen to Ginny F., 39:

"I married my husband when I was 30. He was unbelievably sexy, adventuresome, fun to be with, and I loved him. Then I slowly started to gain weight. He would order special meals before going to work and I spent all day making sure the meal turned out just beautiful. Food is love, right? I had absolutely no concept of a balanced meal and hated green vegetables so I didn't serve them. When I became pregnant, I was scared. Look at all the weight I was going to gain—and I did. After the baby was born I weighed 161. No wonder it was a difficult birth.

"The summer after the baby was born I injured my back and laid on the floor constantly for three months, but I did not stop eating. Up to 175. Hospitalization, and a long recovery followed.

"The next entire year was pure hell. My mother died. I spent three months watching it happen. My little boy was entering the terrible two's. I had to be very careful with my back. My husband was transferred. We had to sell our nice little home. We searched for months before we could find a home we could afford.

"By now my weight was up to 185. I had a hard time recovering from my mother's death and the ordeal of watching her die. I was depressed and upset most of the time. I tried being all the things I should be to fit into the community. Tennis? Swimming? Volunteer hospital work? No, no, no. I was too FAT. I hated myself. About this time an orthopedic surgeon told me I would be a very poor risk on the operating table. That just about did it. I saw no end to my misery. I hurt so bad between being fat and being without direction, I couldn't function properly. It was hard just to be alive. This was the lowest point of my life."

That was the point when Ginny began the program. Then she wrote:

"On the program 3 weeks!

"A crazy thing has happened to me. I feel thin. My mind pictures the girl I was, and I feel just as though I am that girl with a fairly nice figure. I look at my body and see I am still fat BUT now I know I will eventually see the scale catch up with my mind! I enrolled in a college extension course.

"Five weeks on the program.

"I think I have lost about 18 pounds. Amazing, I'm fitting into clothes I haven't worn for three years. Today five separate people complimented me about how nice I looked, including my boss!"

Yes, it was a change in food. But, it was also a change in attitude. Notice there was no bellyaching about problems in her later writing. But of course, her problems were most significant and meaningful to her just as yours are to you.

Problems may not be solved by the One-Day-At-A-Time Plan, but your attitude toward them and yourself will be changed. And that makes a heap of difference in the amount of sun that shines in your day and the amount of weight you lose day by day.

Randy L. had the habit of falling apart when a problem hit. Everything in his life seemed to explode. A few days into the program, though, he noticed a surprising change.

"Today was really a milestone for me. In the past when this kind of crisis arose, I would have bolted, eaten all I could lay my hands on, and gone on a food spending spree. This crisis shook me up, but I just took a long hard look at me. Was I about to indulge in some careless, impulsive action? I watched me. I was in control. This has been really good. I need the confidence that this program has given me."

Confidence gave Randy a better self-image. A better self-image equals a better physical image—slender, attractive, youthful, healthy.

What to Do Before You Begin

I want to review with you the steps you need to take before you begin the One-Day-At-A-Time Plan.

Some of you, I am sure, have already taken these steps. But sometimes you are so anxious to continue reading this book that you do not take all the preparatory actions called for.

Since the notebook you have been asked to prepare is your basic "road map," let's review the steps you need to take from its viewpoint.

1. Prepare the notebook according to the instructions at the beginning of Chapter III.

2. Keep a record of your flour and sugar intake today and a record a week from today. Enter these records on pages 2 and 3. Mark these pages completed by drawing the progress chart line across the title page to the right-hand margin.

3. You are about to cancel a number of foods from your life and substitute others in their place. Again, referring to Chapter III, copy the disallowed foods into your notebook on page 4. Draw the progress lines on the title page toward the right-hand margin in order to "flag" your progress for each "Activity."

4. Write the allowable foods on page 5. "Flag" your progress.

5. Make a record of your present weight at the top of page 6, and your ideal weight at the bottom of the page. You will occasionally be entering your weight and the date on this page.

6. Do the same for your measurements on Page 7.

7. On page 8, make a diary type of entry about how you have been feeling. Be sure to include any ailments that have required ongoing medical treatment. Later, you will be making additional entries on this page to reflect your physical and mental (emotional) health in the days, weeks, and months ahead.

8. Relax and write. If you feel this writing is philosophical and general about life, let it flow on page 9, Meditations. If it is about you and what you think of yourself, write on page 18, Self-Image. If it is a letter to someone, even me, to get something off your chest, write on

page 34, Letters. It is advisable to develop the writing technique before starting the One-Day-At-A-Time Plan.

9. Give yourself mental instructions. Relax and use the words and images (mental pictures) that help switch foods and thoughts. Record the words and images you use on page 26, Subconscious Instructions. Always draw the line farther to the right on the title page opposite the appropriate "Weight Loss Activity" to indicate the progress you have made.

10. Give away sugar, starch, and fatty products. Write how you felt giving them away. Prepare menus. Go shopping for protein and other allowable foods. Place the water jug in your refrigerator. And begin.

The One-Day-At-A-Time Plan Begins— And Overweight Ends

I am saddened to leave you. I will be delighted if you keep me constantly near you. Then you will always have the pages of this book reminding and encouraging you to set and to reach your ultimate goal, day by day.

It has been fun sharing with you what your new, slender, and exciting life can so easily be like—one day at a time.

Allow your daily progress to accelerate and inspire your continuous success—to achieve your miracle.

As you experience your success, share it with others. Your personal triumph can be an inspiration for others who are up in weight and down in mind and in spirits.

You need to pull yourself together to shed the excess pounds day by day, and to make *your* world a happier world in which to live. We all need to pull together day to day to make this a better, happier world to live in.

I am betting that you will enjoy the One-Day-At-A-Time Plan so much that it will become your daily, automatic way of eating, thinking, doing, and being. I am betting that the avalanche of benefits will influence you to avoid fatty items, old sweets, and sticky ways—forever.

I am betting that, in the process, you will meet and understand a wonderful person. This person will evoke your love, admiration, and respect. This person will learn to achieve and to do. This person is the real you.

Enjoy your protein meals and all the delicious, nutritive foods.
Enjoy your relaxation sessions, meditative writings, self-enlightenment; your new outer and inner being.
Enjoy your longer, slender, healthier and happier life—one day at a time.
ENJOY——